# Critical Issues in Youth Work Management

This valuable textbook communicates the complexities and controversies at the heart of youth work management, exploring key issues in a critical fashion. Written by a team of experienced youth work lecturers, the chapters cover topics such as planning, evaluation and supervision, whilst acknowledging the changing structures of integrated services and the impact of public service reform.

Divided into three sections, it covers:

- historical and theoretical context;
- critical practice issues, including leadership, policy constraints, planning and accountability;
- managing in different settings, for instance integrated services and the voluntary sector.

Aimed at both youth work students studying for their professional qualification, as well as practising managers, *Critical Issues in Youth Work Management* encourages critical thinking about what management in youth work is and what it can be. It includes reflective questions and further reading, and case studies are integrated throughout.

**Jon Ord** is Reader in Youth and Community Work at UCP Marjon, Plymouth, UK. He has worked as a youth worker for twenty years, and is the author of *Youth Work Process, Product and Practice*, as well as a number of articles concerning the theory and practice of youth work.

# Critical Issues in Youth Work Management

**Edited by
Jon Ord**

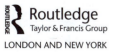 Routledge
Taylor & Francis Group

LONDON AND NEW YORK

First published 2012
by Routledge
2 Park Square, Milton Park, Abingdon, Oxon OX14 4RN

Simultaneously published in the USA and Canada
by Routledge
711 Third Avenue, New York, NY 10017

*Routledge is an imprint of the Taylor & Francis Group, an informa business*

*British Library Cataloguing in Publication Data*
A catalogue record for this book is available from the British Library

*Library of Congress Cataloging-in-Publication Data*
Critical issues in youth work management / edited by Jon Ord. -- 1st ed.
p. cm.
1. Social work with youth--Great Britain. 2. Personnel management--Great Britain.
3. Responsibility. I. Ord, Jon.
HV1441.G7C75 2011
362.7′2530941--dc23
2011019839

ISBN13: 978-0-415-59434-9 (hbk)
ISBN13: 978-0-415-59435-6 (pbk)
ISBN13: 978-0-203-18094-5 (ebk)

Typeset in Times
by Taylor & Francis Books

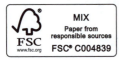

Printed and bound in Great Britain by
TJ International Ltd, Padstow, Cornwall

To Sue, Nathan and Evan


Not everything that can be counted counts and not everything that counts can be counted

(On a wall in Einstein's Princeton office)

# Contents

# List of Figures

# Contributors

**Ilona Buchroth** is a Senior Lecturer in Community and Youth Work at the University of Sunderland. Prior to this she has worked as a community education service manager, youth and community development worker, adult education tutor and teacher. She has a longstanding and active involvement in the voluntary sector.

**Paul Bunyan** is Senior Lecturer in Youth and Community Work at Edge Hill University. His main research interests are around community organizing, civil society and political theory.

**Sue Cooper** is a senior lecturer at the UCP Marjon, Plymouth, on the Youth and Community Work programmes and the M.A. Professional Practice. Her specialisms include management, supervision and evaluation. She joined the team in 2005, leaving a senior management role in Hampshire Youth Service.

**Bernard Davies** has been a youth worker, youth officer and tutor on professional courses. He is a visiting professor at Leicester De Montfort University and chair of 42nd Street, a young people's mental health resource in Manchester. His publications include a three-volume history of the youth service in England.

**Simon Davies** has over ten years experience managing youth and community projects in the faith-based and statutory sectors. He is Senior Lecturer in Youth and Community Work at Youthworks, Oxford, and works in partnership with churches and Christian charities in the professional and theological development of Christian youth workers.

**Pat Fuller** has worked in voluntary and statutory sectors and in paid and voluntary capacities as a manager in: community work in Liverpool and Sunderland, in youth work in Bristol, Liverpool, Durham and Bradford. She is currently a Senior Lecturer in Youth and Community Work at Leeds Metropolitan University

**Pauline Grace** is Senior lecturer and M.A. Co-ordinator of Youth and Community Work at Newman University College, Birmingham. She has over twenty-three years of youth work experience as a front line worker, supervisor, manager and trainer in the West Midlands. She is a member of the campaign 'In Defence of Youth Work'.

**Graham Griffiths** is course leader for the Youth and Community Development programmes at Bradford College. He has worked in both statutory voluntary sectors, and has an interest in residential work. A member of CYWU/Unite, he is committed to anti-oppressive practice and is involved with community groups in his local area.

**Roger Harrison** is a Senior Lecturer in Education at the Open University. His teaching work is developing a programme of courses leading to professional qualification of youth workers. His research is on the discursive formation of professional identities among students and practitioners.

**Sue Lea** has worked in leadership and management roles in retailing, banking, local government, higher education and the voluntary sector for over thirty years. She teaches educational management at undergraduate level, and management and leadership in youth and community work and in the early years at UCP Marjon, Plymouth.

**Bryan Merton** was H. M. Inspector for Schools responsible for youth work and policy until 1996. He has subsequently trained leaders and managers in the sector, conducted research and evaluation, and provided advice to government, local authorities, development agencies and voluntary organizations. He is Visiting Professor at De Montfort University.

**Mohamed Moustakim** is a Programme Leader of the M.A. in Youth and Community Work at the University of East London. He is the British Educational Research Association Convenor of the Youth Studies Special Interest Group. He previously worked as a youth worker.

**Jon Ord** worked as a youth worker for twenty years, and is now a Reader in Youth and Community Work at UCP Marjon, Plymouth. He is the author of the book *Youth Work Process, Product and Practice*, as well as a number of articles concerning the theory and practice of youth work.

**Kate Sapin** has directed programmes in community and youth work at the University of Manchester for over twenty years. Author of *Essential Skills for Youth Work Practice* (Sage, 2009), her particular interests include adult learning, professional supervision, participative and anti-oppressive practice, and the organization and development of community projects.

**Graeme Tiffany** has a background in youth and community work. Now a freelance trainer, lecturer and education consultant, he has special interests in detached and street-based youth work, democratic education and the use of philosophical tools to support learning. Follow his activities and read his blog at www.graemetiffany.co.uk/

**Emily Wood** is currently a Youth Work Manager for Merton Council, a director of Brighton Youth Centre and a trustee and treasurer for the Charlotte Miller Art Project. She has fifteen years of experience of youth work in the UK and internationally, and is a qualified youth worker, with an M.A. from Goldsmiths University.

# Acknowledgements

First I would like to thank Sarah Banks and Tony Jeffs for their advice and support in preparing the initial proposal. Their words: 'you'll only do this once' helped keep me sane and enabled me to realize that this was just the normal process of editing. I would also like to thank Routledge for agreeing to publish the book and for their support during its writing and publication, as well as the anonymous reviewers who helped shape the early structure.

I'd like to thank my colleagues and students at UCP Marjon, discussions with whom have helped shape the thinking behind this book. Thanks are due in particular to Sue Cooper, whose excellent management of the department enables some time and space to be dedicated to research; Sue Lea, who provided considerable support in the early stages of my teaching on the management module at Marjon; and to Christine Smith for her thoughts on managing youth centres, which ought, given a different set of circumstances, to have been translated into a specific contribution.

I must offer a special thanks to the contributors, for their time and commitment and for putting up with my endless requests. This book is a genuine collation of a breadth, and depth, of knowledge, as well as expertise, and is all the better for it.

And finally I would like to thank Dave Williams and Brenda Malloy for those 'first lessons' in youth work; my mother, who enabled me to find my own way; and last but certainly not least, my wife Sue and my two sons Nathan and Evan, for their support during the editorial process – no doubt they will be as glad to see it finally on the shelf as I will …

# Introduction

## *Jon Ord*

This is more than simply a book about management; it is a book which asks critical questions about both what management is, and should be, in youth work. It begins with a thought-provoking reflection upon the historical development of management by Bernard Davies in Chapter 1, demonstrating that the current 'phenomenon' of management is a relatively new concept in the history of youth work, and that management was historically associated with the role of 'advisor' – someone who supported, guided and influenced practice but didn't control it. Importantly, the growth in management coincided with the increased attention paid to youth work by government. However, whilst the current form of management in the public sector, (broadly described as new public management or more pejoratively as 'managerialism'[1]) arrived with Thatcherism, it was not until New Labour paid particular close attention to youth work that managerialism began to bite. This close association between management and policy is perhaps best evidenced in the construction of leadership in youth work. Sue Lea in Chapter 5 makes the case that leadership is almost entirely associated with mobilization of the workforce to deliver an external framework of policy directives, resulting in leaders becoming mere conduits for policymakers.

This book questions the 'taken for granted' notion of management, arguing that rather than 'value free', management is necessarily 'value laden'. The current form of management presents itself as value neutral, with its emphasis upon the apparently objective striving for greater efficiency and effectiveness. However, the values which underpin this form of management in youth work, it is argued, are fundamentally neoliberal, with an emphasis on the private over public sector and the pre-eminence of the market. This is explored in some depth in Chapter 2, which charts the shift from welfarism, associated with social democracy, to post welfarism, which is underpinned by neoliberalism. It makes comparisons between New Labour and Thatcher's more strident neoliberalism, and whilst it is acknowledged there are elements of the social democratic tradition within New Labour, ultimately it is the neoliberal which dominates. The last chapter of the first section of the book, which characterizes the 'context of youth work management', looks at the competing 'theories' underpinning management. Initially it looks at the relative merits of mainstream or modernist management, before introducing post-modern management, and exploring the dominant discourse of management, which creates a straitjacket of technical rationalism underpinned by the discipline of auditing and accountability.

The second part of the book, entitled 'Critical issues in the practice of youth work management', assesses the impact of new public management or managerialism on the management of youth work. It begins by introducing labour process theory, which argues that dissent is a consequence of disempowerment, and structural inequality, and therefore is not something which should be managed out, but contains legitimate concerns which should be incorporated into the managerial process. It then goes on to argue, with reference to literature from critical management studies, that disparate voices are too often silenced by current management practices, and they to need to be incorporated. The question of what are the appropriate structures and cultures for youth work management is then asked, concluding that if youth work is to be consistent with its own values, it must make a commitment to democracy, at the heart of its managerial processes.

Chapters 6 and 7 in this part focus on planning and evaluation; both chapters criticize the emphasis on objective and quantifiable measures in youth work, arguing that in relation to planning, it is not only untenable but counter-productive to try to tie youth workers' planning to specific outcomes prior to the engagement of youth people and the development of a process of youth work. In relation to evaluation, Sue Cooper argues that the concept of quality is essentially subjective and as a result participative approaches must be re-emphasized, which gives voice to practitioners and young people. This section continues with an analysis of the impact of managerialism on centre-based youth work management, looking at the involvement of young people, the impact of targets and programming, and health and safety. It argues that not only are youth centre managers spending increasingly less time delivering face-to-face work, but the community context has been eroded. Graeme Tiffany's final chapter in this section offers a critique of detached youth work management, arguing that it needs to be 'intelligence based', i.e. involve a bottom-up process grounded in information elicited from contact with young people, rather than a top-down imposition of a set of outcomes designated for young people independent of any genuine needs analysis.

The final part of the book looks at three important settings of youth work management, namely integrated services, the faith-based sector, and the voluntary sector. Merton and Davies' chapter draws together key lessons from their recent research into the impact of integrated services on youth work management. Their tentative conclusions suggest a disparity between practitioners' sceptical views of the success of integrated services and those of managers which appeared more positive; as well as increased uncertainty and complexity. Simon Davies' faith-based chapter focuses on management in Christian youth work. This offers a different set of challenges, not least because managerialism has had very little, if any, impact. Faith-based youth work management is more reminiscent of the era of 'youth advisor'. The creation of vocationally driven 'lone rangers' is perhaps an issue which needs to be addressed, but it does offer up a mirror to challenge the managerialist practices of secular youth work management.

The final chapter of the book is an important assessment of the impact of managerialism on the voluntary sector, as well as an analysis of the possibilities of the 'Big Society'. It charts the changing face of the voluntary sector with the impact of the new accountability – how funding patterns have shifted, the effect of the contract culture, and how the locus of control has shifted from local communities to the state. It also assesses the sustainability of the voluntary sector due to the increase in short termism, and competition between providers. It concludes that in theory at least the Big Society embraces a vibrant voluntary sector, but in reality unless sufficient support is given to the sector it is hard to see it as anything more than a smokescreen for an ideological assault on welfarism.

It is hoped that this book will give readers the opportunity to reflect upon the growth of management in youth work, and gain a deeper of understanding of the impact of managerial practices, as well as see management from a different, more critical, perspective. It is argued that the current managerial practices are neither necessary, nor inevitable. Furthermore, and perhaps more importantly despite witnessing the rise of managerialism, we may now (assisted in part by the cuts to the tier of management itself) begin to challenge its dominance. It is also hoped that this book will play a part in assisting both practitioners and managers alike to begin to develop managerial practices which are consistent with the values and practices of youth work, not least of which is the importance of democracy.

## Note

1 'managerialism is a set of beliefs and practices, the core of which burns the seldom tested assumption that better management will prove an effective solvent for a wide range of economic and social ills' (Pollitt, C., 1993, *Managerialism and the Public Services*, 2nd edn, Oxford: Blackwell, p. 1).

# Part I

# The context of youth work management

# 1 From advice to management

## The arrival of youth workers' accountability

*Bernard Davies*

Over the past fifty years the title of those with organizational oversight of youth work has mutated from 'organizer' and 'advisor' to 'officer' and 'manager'. This, however, has represented much more than a change of name. When the state 'service of youth' was created in 1939 the role's main priorities were support and advice for field practitioners operating with considerable discretion and autonomy. By the later 1990s, Blairite New Public Management (NPM) had increasingly required the role to exercise top-down direction and control of 'delivery' focused on tightly defined value-for-money social objectives. This chapter traces how these changes have also brought a fundamental cultural shift in how youth work practice is conceived and carried out.

### When good intentions were enough …

Although this is not a piece about a lost golden age, it starts with a youth worker practising throughout the 'swinging' sixties and into the 1970s. He'd been brought up on a then still-emerging version of professionalism which implicitly said: 'As long as your values and goals are right, then all will be well'. Implicit, too, was the message: 'And because you articulate your intentions as young people-focused and about their needs, you don't need to explain how far you are actually achieving them'. 'Outcomes', insofar as these were ever considered, would, it was assumed, take care of themselves, leaving accountability, at best, an intuitive and unarticulated process.

In caricatured form, the youth worker here was me. Nor apparently was what I recall just a figment of my failing memory. In 1988 Jeffs and Smith talked of youth work's occupational culture as imbued with:

> a deep-seated resistance to 'being told what to do'. Something of the frontier spirit remains, with the lone cowboy or cowgirl … simply going where the trail takes them.
>
> (1988: 236)

While acknowledging that this could lead to 'a rich diversity of practice', they concluded that youth work was 'still perceived as offering the opportunity to maximise freedom and minimalise accountability' (Jeffs and Smith, 1988: 236). Moreover, this resistance to being accountable for what the practice was achieving did not just apply to policy-makers' and funders' expectations. Little systematic attention was given to checking 'impact' on the purported beneficiaries of the work – young people and their communities. For this absence of mind, youth work and its practitioners were eventually to pay a high price.

## The youth officer as organizer, advisor and administrator

If this was how workers were then operating, how did 'management' manage them? How far did tackling the dominant youth worker approach to the work appear in managers' job descriptions (where these existed) or in their understanding of the role?

Even before a state 'Service of Youth' was created in 1939 (see below), national voluntary organizations were increasingly employing 'field officers' and 'specialist advisers' to help plan and improve local youth club provision and train leaders (see Henriques, 1934: 232; 1951: viii). This did not, however, involve directly 'managing' clubs (all of which were independent) or their staff (who were anyway overwhelmingly voluntary). Primarily the job was advisory and administrative.

Moreover, bureaucratic notions of 'management' sat uncomfortably with the assumptions, deeply rooted in organizations so overwhelmingly reliant on volunteers, that 'youth leadership' was a vocation (see Jeffs, 2006) and that those who took on the role could therefore be trusted to carry it out without close scrutiny. Formalized accountability procedures were thus irrelevant – even demeaning. Indeed, often the problem was that workers, including the small number of full-time paid workers, did whatever was needed to fulfil their vocational 'mission', no matter how many hours this took. Such over-commitment did not of course guarantee *quality*. It did, though, make it harder for a 'youth advisor' or even a club management committee to hold a worker openly accountable or even to recognize this was needed.

During and after the 1914–18 war a small number of local authorities had offered funding to the voluntary youth sector (Jeffs, 1979: 13). However, the most significant shift came in 1939 with the release of Circular 1486, 'The Service of Youth' (Board of Education, 1939), with annual grants which 'made it possible for field officers to be appointed to expand and develop their work' (Evans, 1965: 23). These 'servants' of the voluntary organizations also increasingly found themselves working alongside local education authority youth officers whose numbers grew significantly (ibid.). With some of the new LEA youth organizers coming directly from the voluntary sector, many of its assumptions and approaches were carried over into statutory services (Percival, 1951: 169), including a light-touch support and advisory style in their approach to club workers. Writing in 1943 for 'those who have responded to the call of Circular 1486', Desirée Edward-Rees – herself a West Riding of Yorkshire youth officer – noted that:

> Most Education Authorities now employ organisers, or officers, to administer the work of their Central Youth Committee and to advise their local youth councils.
>
> (1943: 118)

Emerging as it did out of a war against ruthless totalitarian regimes, the new Youth Service had to contend with 'a very real and genuine fear of anything modelled on the continental Youth Movements' (Macalister Brew, 1943: 25). One of the early challenges for this new breed of youth officer was to deal with the perception of them as *state* officials. State papers themselves displayed considerable sensitivity to this, with the second major war-time Circular on the Service of Youth (1516) proclaiming that 'any attempt at a State-controlled uniformity or regimentation would be both stupid and perilous ... ' The function of the state it saw as 'to supplement the resources of existing national organizations without impairing their independence ... ' (Board of Education, 1940, cited in Davies, 1999: 20).

Macalister Brew, though warmly welcoming the appearance of the new youth officer posts, nonetheless echoed these concerns, regretting that they were labelled 'youth organizer' as this was 'so reminiscent of Nazism and Fascism' (1943: 34). For Gordon Ette, Youth Officer for Wolverhampton and treasurer of the National Conference of Youth Service Officers founded in 1940 (Roberts, 1944: 56), the worry was more pragmatic – that: 'The danger inherent in the new set-up is that the service will be cluttered with an increasing army of organizers who want to centralize everything' (Ette, 1949: 118). As late as 1960, two officers of the National Association of Youth Leaders and Organizers (NAYLO) were still referring to the danger of 'a state-run youth movement' (*Times Education Supplement*, 1960). Circular 1516 made this more explicit, and the mirror image of these anxieties was a sensitivity about relations with the still highly influential voluntary youth organizations – the local and regional embodiments of the Scouts and Guides, the various Brigades, boys, girls and mixed clubs' associations and what would now be termed 'faith-based' organizations. Circular 1486 was unambiguous that in the new local youth committees:

> The individual traditions and special experience of youth possessed by the voluntary organizations will be joined by the prestige and resources of the local education authority.
>
> (Board of Education, 1939: para. 8)

Ette thus emphasized that 'a wisely planned local youth service' will recognize these organizations' distinctive features (1939: 120). For Macalister Brew this meant that the youth officer's first task was 'to help and encourage all the voluntary organizations to fit into the (local authority) plan' (1943: 25, 38). The new youth officers' core tasks thus remained much as they had been for their voluntary organization predecessors: organizing to provide, but not directly manage, practical and financial resources and support those working face-to-face with young people. Over the following decade little apparently changed. By 1954 Peter Keunstler, in again highlighting 'the important role played by youth officers and others', did choose to stress 'a happy relationship between the authorities and youth workers generally' (1954: 43). On the other hand, Macalister Brew's chapter on management, helpers' and members' committees in her influential book *Youth and Youth Groups* made no mention of the new breed of statutory youth officers (1957: 184–99).

The Albemarle Report, published in 1960, gave strong endorsement to these posts: after noting that 'there are still authorities ... who have no Youth Service officer or equivalent post', it concluded: 'We find it hard to see how such an authority can properly carry out its obligations under the [Education] Act'. However, it continued to bracket organizers and officers with both voluntary bodies and local education authorities, whilst still describing the latter as responsible for 'the proper servicing of youth groups in the area' through for example 'information and advice'; for assessing youth groups' need for premises and equipment; and for organizing 'common services', particularly training (Ministry of Education, 1960: 84–85).

Albemarle did, however, advocate that the youth officer move beyond purely 'administrative' functions so that 'his primary task' came to be seen as that of 'field-worker'. It also implied that the role should shift towards managing staff as this might be understood today – that for example the youth officer 'must know his youth groups and be able to assess their achievement and to help them improve it'. It also insisted that 'the supervision and guidance of leaders ... is his responsibility' (Ministry of Education, 1960: 85).

A decade later, the Fairbairn-Milson report (DES, 1969: 120), while noting that 'the status of the Youth Officer (or equivalent) varies widely', sought mainly to bend the role to its own often conflicting priorities. To underpin the Fairbairn sub-committee's aim of locating youth work with younger age groups within schools, it reaffirmed their historic function by suggesting that youth officers act as advisers in social education alongside other school advisers (1969: 123). By contrast, to support the Milson sub-committee's preoccupation with community development approaches for the 16-pluses, it recommended their work be linked to – even perhaps be merged into – that of the new town corporations' 'social relations officers' (1969: 126).

For other commentators, staff accountability still did not merit any explicit consideration. Though Davies and Gibson (1967: 148–49) emphasized the 'sanctions' on youth work practice which emanate from 'society' (which could include 'sponsors') and from young people, their section on 'management' (1967: 197–201) made no reference to accountability. The definition of their role by the youth officers' own professional body (then termed: National Association of Youth Service Officers) still emphasized 'close liaison' with the voluntary organizations and an ability 'to advise on all matters effecting the Youth Service including the forms of aid available through the LEA' (Leicester and Farndale, 1967: 224).

Four years later John Leigh did acknowledge that some youth officers were by then making 'an enormous number of "decisions" in the sense of interpretations of aims' and that these 'to a large extent affect the practice of the service' (1971: 28–29). Nonetheless, for him the role's priorities continued to be:

> the siting of clubs and their staffing and equipment, the kinds of in-service and part-time worker training which are appropriate and the various supporting services to be made available to the youth clubs.
>
> (Ibid.)

## The youth officer as supervisor

This conception of the youth officer's role as primarily 'advisory' persisted in places into the 1980s, for example as late as 1987–88 Sheffield Youth Service's principal officer was still a member of the education department's advisory team. However, by the late 1960s the rapid increase in the number of newly qualified workers (from the 700 Albemarle identified in the late 1950s to 1,550 by 1968; Davies, 1999: 64–65) brought new expectations of the youth officer's role, central to which was 'supervision', especially for newly appointed staff, as had been advocated by the Albemarle Report.

Even so, in calling as early as 1962 for 'the supervision of the new recruit', the principal of the National College for the Training of Youth Leaders, Edward Sidebottom, was still insisting that this:

is not just a question of administrative control: it involves the provision of good counsel and sometimes simply ... a 'sounding board' for the leader.

(Sidebottom, 1962)

Although this was seen as 'not *just* a question of administrative control' it perhaps indicated a shift in thinking. The following year Sidebottom again advocated 'proper supervisory help' to enable 'rapid progression in the work of the new leader', suggesting there was 'a strong case for running some short courses in supervisory methods and for the publication of some helpful literature' (Sidebottom, 1963). By the end of the decade, both had been achieved. In 1967 Joan Tash gave a detailed account of a two-year project for training youth workers in the skills of supervision – where 'supervision' meant discussions between a youth worker and 'another person who had no authority over him [sic.]' (1967: 9). Nonetheless, with the report demonstrating how such 'non-managerial' supervision could help workers perform to their potential and develop professionally, its approach was seen, too, as relevant to what became known as 'managerial supervision'.

Meanwhile, in 1966, the Department of Education and Science (DES) sponsored the first of two courses for 60 Youth Service Officers. The second in 1968–69, attended by 45 men and 12 women, 39 of whom were from the statutory sector (Gibson, 1970: 8), revealed a growing concern about managerial supervision, with one whole section of the syllabus aiming: 'to help Youth Officers to practise a supervisory function that will encourage the growth and development of the staff whom they lead' (Gibson, 1970: 19). Although the evidence only emerged later, there had clearly been a need for such training. As a report, published in 1972 on the work of the National College between 1961 and 1970, noted: 'the need for supervision, particularly during the first year of full-time work, has been recognised for some time. The problem has been to supply it' (Watkins 1972: 109).

Responses from past National College students revealed that, though the proportions were increasing, only 40 per cent of 1969 graduates saw themselves as being supervised and only about 30 per cent rated their supervision as satisfactory (ibid.). By then the youth workers' own professional body, the Youth Service Association (YSA) was also running courses in supervision. As well as filling a support gap for new entrants, such supervision also has to be seen in the context of the wider struggle to establish youth work's credentials as a professional occupation requiring carefully nurtured specialist expertise. No doubt unintentionally, in the name of 'professional autonomy' and 'professional discretion', the claim to professional status in effect provided an up-dated rationale for that 'deep-seated resistance to being told what to do' (Jeffs and Smith, 1988: 230), thus further reinforcing the predominantly non-directive styles of 'oversight' inherited from the voluntary sector.

## State intervention and the pressure to manage

However, as exemplified and reinforced by the Albemarle report, the balance was tipping away from the post-war fear of a state-run youth movement to an openness to – even a demand for – a more proactive state role in youth work provision. In 1968 this was made explicit by a forthright leading article in *Youth Review* – the magazine jointly sponsored by the National Association of Youth Service Officers (NAYSO) and the YSA – which argued: 'what the Youth Service needs now is a proper plan – Authoritative guidance – a directive' (*Youth Review*, 1968: 3). The following year, the Rev. Roy Herbert talked of 'a failure to face the need for some nationally accepted yardstick by which to judge (youth work) standards' (1969: 3), while ten years later participants at a conference of the Community and Youth Service Association (CYSA, formerly the YSA) were calling for a definition and delineation of the government's 'core responsibilities and of its area of work/influence' (see Davies, 1978b: 11).

However, these advocates of stronger and clearer *state* leadership seemed never quite to address the crucial accountability questions left hanging throughout youth work's earlier laissez-faire period. Who would ensure the government lead was followed? Who would set the standards for which Herbert had called? Who would judge if they were being met – and how? How sensitive such 'managerial' questions could be was illustrated by a sharp debate stirred up in 1967 by a county youth officer's suggestion that youth work professionalism needed to be shaped by 'a simple pattern of management activity' involving 'setting goals', 'determining operations', 'determining resources' and 'creating conditions [including] … the disciplines which will need to be observed to avoid wasting human and material resources' (Bourne, 1967).

During the 1970s, pressure of this kind to redefine the youth officer's role began to build, receiving official if indirect endorsement in the second youth officers' course programme, mentioned above. This for example proposed that youth officers should be supported:

> Especially by helping them in the managerial part of their work and by considering what parts of the knowledge and experience of the functioning and management of industrial and commercial organizations would be relevant and useful to them.
>
> (Gibson, 1970: 19)

Moreover, an analysis of the pre-course experience of the ten National College student cohorts of the 1960s also suggested that some of youth workers' own perspectives on their engagement with their organizations was evidence of a burgeoning worker/manager divide. Youth workers appeared to have a growing perception of themselves *as* 'workers' evidenced by the expression of one worker in 1972: 'Don't join the professionals: that would kill youth work' (Hamilton, 1972: 13–15). Interestingly, of those who by the early 1970s had become youth officers, only 25 per cent had previously been in working-class occupations, with 80 per cent from working-class backgrounds remaining in face-to-face practice (Watkins, 1972: 81). Increasingly field practitioners began to distinguish themselves, and their roles, from those to whom they were answerable. The existence of a 'worker/manager' divide was further confirmed in 1983 by the conversion of their professional association, CYSA, into a trade union – the Community and Youth Workers Union (CYWU), albeit only after agonized debates (Davies, 1988; Nichols, 2009).

## The arrival of management and external accountability

The crucial break with past notions of the youth officer's role, and the arrival of explicitly hierarchical notions of 'management', as well as 'managing for accountability' were precipitated by fundamental shifts in the wider political, economic circumstances. Even during the 1960s commentators were warning that existing levels of increase in public expenditure were damaging 'economic progress' (see for example Jay,

1967; Glennerster, 1976: 252–53). But by the early 1970s, these limits became all too real as the 'never-had-it-so-good' times of the 1960s evaporated in the heat of huge oil price increases, destabilizing balance-of-payments crises and ruthless International Monetary Fund interventions in the British economy. The resultant financial 'stringency' within the public sector brought increasingly tight control of the use of its resources.

These trends were underpinned in 1974 by local government reorganization resulting in many local authorities adopting the procedures of corporate management (see Benington, 1976) which required local government officers to operate as managers responsible for calling staff to account. By 1977 a 'great education debate' was also under way which in effect insisted that training for the economy came first, learning for personal development a poor second. Here too, it was assumed, managers delegated to implement those policies would be less tolerant of the 'frontier spirit' style still entrenched in youth work's occupational culture.

Explicit confirmation of this changed environment came from one senior DES civil servant in 1978. In a note to the Youth Service Forum, the government's youth work consultative body, Barney Baker 'pose[d] fundamental questions about the justification of present practice and the needs of the adolescent' (1978: 1). These he explored both in this paper and in a presentation to a joint annual conference of the CYSA and the National Association of Youth and Community Education Officers (NAYCEO, formerly NAYSO). This in itself indicated that workers and managers were not yet seeing their occupational interests as intrinsically divided.

Baker's conclusions were to have profound and long-term consequences, not just for Youth Service policy but also for how the management of youth work was to develop. One was that 'an assessment of needs in relation to society's … interests' had by then become a priority. Second was that these interests 'may be defined in terms more or less unpalatable to young people'. Finally, Baker urged that the forum 'should make the case for expenditure on the Youth Service principally by reference to the social objectives which it serves' (1978: 5–6). Ensuring that these wider societal, including financial, objectives were being met implied that youth workers would have to account for what they did in much clearer and more systemic ways. As another contributor to the CYSA-NAYCEO conference pointed out:

> The day of the free-wheeling, spontaneous, maverick practitioner who went out and did his [sic.] innovating thing … has largely gone. Today, I believe, we are almost all functionaries for some large-scale administrative machine, in which decisions are normally made 'at the top', some distance from where the action is and often according to management criteria like cost-effectiveness.
>
> (Davies, 1978a: 12)

It was in this new climate that the consequences of youth work's past failure to grasp the accountability nettle caught up with it. Already, during the 1970s, through a series of 'black papers', 'the new right' was actively campaigning for a return to traditional ways of measuring the value of education generally (see for example Cox and Boyson, 1977). Increasingly, it became clear, the door had been left open for others to define both the criteria for assessing youth workers' effectiveness – and for doing this in ways which took little account of the distinctive features of their practice. Equally importantly it placed the role of the manager centrally in ensuring this effectiveness.

## Preparing the ground for new public management

The ground was thus well prepared for Margaret Thatcher's post-1979 public sector 'reforms' with their explicit mission to change fundamentally not only the operation of the British welfare state but – even more significantly – the social and cultural assumptions on which it had rested since 1945. During her time in office she kept under repeated pressure those 'woolly liberals' (like youth workers) who continued to adhere to what she saw as the 1960s 'permissive' values and the newly fashionable notion of 'political correctness'. Her targets included professional groups much more powerful and entrenched than youth workers whose powers she and her cabinet colleagues saw as major barriers to providing responsive and 'cost-effective' public services (*Guardian*, 1983).

As secretary of state for education in the early 1970s, Thatcher had taken one of the first steps to requiring youth workers to target their practice, proposing that 'the needs of young school leavers in deprived areas should have special attention' (DES, 1971). Subsequent Labour governments built on these expectations, suggesting in 1975 that youth services, as well as catering for 'the needs of the disadvantaged', should also 'take account of the special needs of ethnic minorities' (DES, 1975: paras 5–6). By 1982 Keith Joseph, Thatcher's education secretary, was urging that the 'resources and skills of the Youth Service ... be made available to and incorporated into Youth Training Schemes (YTS)' with the aim very specifically of catering for the young unemployed (DES, 1982a: 7). Two years later, while reiterating the need for these contributions to YTS, he was also pressing local authorities to concentrate on young people with 'special needs' even if this meant allocating relatively fewer resources to other groups (DES, 1984: para. 9).

All this had clear implications for the management of local authority youth services. These policies at least implied that more effort was needed to check whether (even to ensure that) staff were meeting the new requirements – something which the Thompson Review of the Youth Service in England, carried out in 1981–82, identified as needing specific attention. Though subsequently regarded as naively over-simplified, its starting premise was that 'there is no real mystery about good management' which, it asserted, had 'four basic aspects': 'defining objectives, assigning roles, allocating resources and monitoring performance' (DES, 1982b: 74). Seeing it as 'essential that the performance of the local system should be continuously monitored' (DES, 1982b: 79), it therefore encouraged that those on the front line be kept on a much tighter rein.

Indeed, with the need for accountability procedures being increasingly recognized, youth officers were now re-conceptualized as 'managers'. Publications appeared with titles like *Management and Evaluation: A Selective Bibliography for Managers of the Youth Service* (Marken, 1984) and *A Guide to Performance Appraisal* (Rogers, 1987). By 1989–90 an HMI report focused specifically on 'the efficient and effective management of youth work' was concluding that 'managers are becoming increasingly clear about the purpose of the work and target groups to be served', with the Youth Service 'beginning to develop management systems ... which can help in judgements about performance' (DES, 1991a: 1).

The final piece of the pre-New Labour management jigsaw also appeared in 1991: the report of another Youth Service review whose title (*Managing the Youth Service in the 1990s*) and whose provenance (the business consultancy firm Coopers and Lybrand Deloitte) was clearly indicative of the value placed upon the private sector. One of the four key issues highlighted by the report was 'quality assurance' – itself a relatively new injection into the youth work discourse – about which it drew three subsequently highly influential conclusions – that:

> Current monitoring and evaluation of youth work is insufficiently robust …
>
> Youth Service managers should expect to take on greater responsibilities for inspections and advice …
>
> The service needs performance indicators at all levels.
>
> (DES, 1991b: paras 20–22)

By the time New Labour came to power in 1997 the foundations had thus been firmly laid for NPM's accountability systems, procedures and processes through which a highly centralizing government could seek to hold public services, including youth work, accountable.

## Conclusion

As we shall see in the following chapter, the managerialist grip on youth work tightened considerably under New Labour. In turn this philosophy and approach attracted considerable criticism from field practitioners and some managers (Spence and Devanney, 2006; Ord, 2007; Davies and Merton, 2009; 2010; IDYW 2010). These criticisms particularly focused on a perceived lack of congruence between many of the defining features of youth work and some of NPM's core assumptions. On the one hand practitioners continued to emphasize young people's *voluntary* engagement and the interests and concerns *they* identified through the negotiation of trusting relationships, as the basis for youth work's educational interventions (Davies, 2005). By contrast managers found themselves under policy pressure to target pre-labelled sections of the youth population whose needs had broadly been defined in advance, with 'outcomes' measured by 'hard' data, often within short time frames; epitomized by the Transforming Youth Work agenda (DfES, 2001, 2002). However, many of these criticisms, although deeply felt, were largely 'a-historical'. Yet, as has been demonstrated, NPM represented a distinct break with a very different and long-established management tradition which, though often too loosely delineated, had been much more in tune with youth work's young people-centred and democratic approaches. The break with the past had therefore been about much more than a change in methodology. It had been cultural too, involving a fundamental challenge to some of the practice's core ways of working.

Thus, policy-makers' increasing insistence from the 1970s on measuring and controlling practice, significantly reduced the youth officer's advisory and support roles (see Davies and Merton, 2009: 39–40). This not only relegated the interpretations of young people's needs by those in closest touch with them, the face-to-face practitioners; it also fundamentally contradicted the very nature of youth work. Though requiring workers to intervene with 'a prepared mind', their practice's intrinsic informality, spontaneity and responsiveness to events as they unfold did not sit comfortably with the inflexibilities of such bureaucratic oversight and constraint. Even if desirable, a wholesale nostalgic return to the past is clearly unlikely, especially in a period of severe financial stringency. However, as Gill Millar concluded from her inquiry into how youth work was being managed in the later 2000s:

[it] cannot simply import management models from other industries, or even from other parts of the public sector. In order to manage youth work well, managers need to be aware of, and work with, the occupational culture.

(2010: 144)

Such awareness would be considerably sharpened if it included a recognition of an older youth work tradition of management shaped by the distinguishing features of the practice and framed by a respect for workers' integrity and autonomy in delivering it.

## Questions for reflection and discussion

1   What's in a name? Reflect on the possible differences between 'youth organizer', 'youth adviser', 'youth officer' and 'senior manager'. What might these differences tell us about the role and function of the youth work manager?
2   How has the notion of accountability altered throughout the history of youth work? To whom are youth workers now accountable? How do they demonstrate that accountability? Given the lessons from history, how 'should' they be accountable?

## Further reading

Davies, B. (1979) 'From social education to social and life skills training: in whose interest?' Available at www.infed.org/archives/bernard_davies/davies_in_whose_interests.htm
——(1999) *From Voluntaryism to Welfare State: A History of the Youth Service in England Vol 1*, Leicester: Youth Work Press, chapter 7.
——(1999) *From Thatcherism to New Labour: A History of the Youth Service in England Vol 2*, Leicester: Youth Work Press, chapters 5 and 7.
Jeffs, T. and Smith, M. K. (1988) 'The promise of management for youth work', in Jeffs, T. and Smith, M. K. (eds) *Welfare and Youth Work Practice*, Basingstoke and London: Macmillan, pp. 230–51.

## References

Baker, B. (1978) 'Youth Service Forum for England and Wales – the future role of the youth service: note by the Secretary', London: Department of Education and Science.
Benington, J. (1976) *Local Government Becomes Big Business*, London: Community Development Projects Information and Intelligence Unit.
Board of Education (1939) *The Service of Youth (Circular 1486)*, London: Board of Education.
——(1940) *The Challenge of Youth (Circular 1516)*, London: Board of Education.
Bourne, E. (1967) 'The unprofessional youth service', *New Society*, 7 December.
Cox, C. B. and Boyson, R. (eds) (1977) *Black Paper 1977*, London: Temple Smith.
Davies, B. (1978a) *Priorities in the Youth and Community Service*, Leicester: National Youth Bureau.
——(1978b) 'Policies for youth into the eighties', *Rapport*, September, p. 11.
——(1981) *The State We're in: Restructuring Youth Policies in Britain*, Leicester: National Youth Agency.
——(1988) 'Professionalism or trade unionism? The search for a collective identity', in Jeffs, T. and Smith, M. (eds) *Welfare and Youth Work Practice*, Basingstoke and London: Macmillan, pp. 200–214.
——(1999) *From Voluntaryism to Welfare State: A History of the Youth Service in England 1939–1979*, Leicester: Youth Work Press.

——(2005) 'Youth work: a manifesto for our times', *Youth and Policy*, no. 88, Summer, pp. 5–27.

Davies, B. and Gibson, A. (1967) *The Social Education of the Adolescent*, London: University of London Press.

Davies, B. and Merton, B. (2009) *Squaring the Circle: Findings of a 'Modest' Inquiry into the State of Youth Work Practice in a Changing Policy Environment*, De Montfort University, available at www.dmu.ac.uk/Images/Squaring%20the%20Circle_tcm6–50166.pdf

——(2010) *Straws in the Wind: The State of Youth Work Practice in a Changing Policy Environment – Phase 2*, De Montfort University.

DES (1969) *Youth and Community Work in the 70s (Milson-Fairbairn Report)*, London: HMSO.

——(1971) *Government Statement on the Youth Service*, London: HMSO.

——(1975) 'Provision for Youth – A Discussion Paper', London: HMSO.

——(1982a) 'The Youth Training Scheme: implications for the education service (Circular 6/82)', London: DES.

——(1982b) *Experience and Participation: Report of the Review Group on the Youth Service in England (Thompson Report)*, London: HMSO.

——(1984) 'Draft circular to all local education authorities and national voluntary youth organisations', London: HMSO.

——(1991a) *Efficient and Effective Management of Youth Work: A Report by HMI*, London: HMSO.

——(1991b) *Managing the Youth Service in the 1990s*, London, HMSO.

DfES (2001) *Transforming Youth Work: Developing Youth Work for Young People*, London: HMSO.

——(2002) *Transforming Youth Work: Resourcing Excellent Youth Services*, London: HMSO.

Edward-Rees, D. (1943) *The Service of Youth Book*, London: The National Society/Society for Promoting Christian Knowledge.

Ette, G. (1949) *For Youth Only*, London: Faber and Faber.

Evans, W. M. (1965) *Young People in Society*, Oxford: Blackwell.

Gibson, A. (1970) *The Youth Service Officers' Course 1968–69: Record of an Experimental Approach to In-Service Training*, Leicester: Youth Service Information Centre.

Glennerster, H. (1976) 'In praise of public expenditure', *New Statesman*, 27 February.

*Guardian* (1983) 'Thatcher team plot their future for the family', 17 February.

Hamilton, R. (1972) 'Don't join the professionals: that would kill youth work', *Youth Review*, no. 25, Winter, 13–14.

Henriques, B. (1934) *Club Leadership*, London: Oxford University Press.

——(1951) *Club Leadership Today*, London: Oxford University Press.

Herbert, R. (1969) *Youth Service – Has It a Future?* London: Church of England Youth Council

IDYW (2010) 'What we stand for', *The* In Defence of Youth Work *Home Page*, www.indefenceofyouthwork.org.uk/wordpress/, accessed 19 April 2010.

Jay, D. (1967) 'Social services – a 70s crisis?' *The Times*, 31 May.

Jeffs, T. (1979) *Young People and the Youth Service*, London: Routledge.

——(2006) 'Too few, too many: the retreat from vocation and calling', *The* Informal Education *Homepage*, www.infed.org/talkingpoint/retreat_from_calling_and_vocation.htm, accessed 29 April 2010.

Jeffs, T. and Smith, M. (1988) 'The promise of management for youth work', in Jeffs, T. and Smith, M. (eds) *Welfare and Youth Work Practice*, Basingstoke: Macmillan, pp. 230–51.

Keunstler, P. (1954) *Youth Work in England*, London: University of London Press.

King George Jubilee Trust (1951) *Youth Service To-morrow*, London: King George Jubilee Trust.

Leicester, J. H. and Farndale, J. (eds) (1967) *Trends in the Services for Youth*, Oxford: Pergamon Press.

Leigh, J. (1971) *Young People and Leisure*, London: Routledge.

Macalister Brew, J. (1943) *In the Service of Youth*, London: Faber and Faber.

——(1957) *Youth and Youth Groups*, London: Faber and Faber.

Marken, M. (1984) *Management and Evaluation: A Selective Bibliography for Managers of the Youth Service*, Leicester: National Youth Bureau.

Millar, G. (2010) 'Managing and developing youth work', in Jeffs, T. and Smith, M. (eds) *Youth Work Practice*, Basingstoke: Palgrave Macmillan, pp. 133–144.

Ministry of Education (1960) *The Youth Service in England and Wales* (Albemarle Report), London: HMSO.

Nichols, D. (2009) *Building Rapport: A Brief History of the Community and Youth Workers Union*, London: Unite the Union.

NYA (2001) *Ethical Conduct in Youth Work: Statement of Values and Principles from the National Youth Agency*, Leicester: NYA.

Ord, J. (2007) *Youth Work Process, Product and Practice: Creating an Authentic Curriculum in Work with Young People*, Lyme Regis: RHP.

Percival, A. C. (1951) *Youth Will Be Led: The Story of the Voluntary Youth Organisations*, London: Collins

Roberts, E. E. (1944) 'The National Conference of Youth Service Officers', in Cooke, D. (ed.) *Youth Organisation of Great Britain 1944–45*, London: Jordan and Sons, pp. 56–59.

Rogers, A. (1987) *A Guide to Performance Appraisal*, Leicester: National Youth Bureau.

Sidebottom, E. (1962) *Further Training for Full-Time Youth Workers*, Leicester: National College for the Training of Youth Leaders.

——(1963) 'Making the best use of professional skill: address to the Youth Service Association', Youth Service Association.

Spence, J. and Devanney, C. (2006) *Youth Work: Voices of Practice*, Leicester: National Youth Agency.

Tash, J. (1967) *Supervision in Youth Work*, London: National Council of Social Service.

*Times Education Supplement* (1960) 'Albemarle Report', 3 March 1960.

Watkins, O. (1972) *Professional Training for Youth Work*, Leicester: Youth Service Information Centre.

*Youth Review* (1968) 'The baby and the bath water', no. 11, Spring.

# 2 The neoliberal policy context of youth work management

## Paul Bunyan and Jon Ord

We saw in the previous chapter how the concept of 'manager' is a relatively recent incarnation in youth work and how it has developed from its predecessor, the 'advisor'. Importantly we also saw how the emergence of the notion of management in youth work was as a direct consequence of specific policy interventions and directives which were shaping youth work practice. The intention in this chapter is to explore more fully the policy context out of which youth work management has evolved.

Youth work has always been shaped by its wider social, political and economic context. It is important therefore that any critical analysis of youth work management is also understood within this context. For over three decades, neoliberalism has constituted the dominant ideological framework through which social policy and the design and delivery of public services has been shaped. Whilst a more strident form of neoliberalism advocated by Thatcher in the 1980s was tempered somewhat by New Labour's 'Third Way', it will be argued the fundamentals remained. These included a preference for 'private' over 'public' sector, and a belief in the importance of a market in delivering a quality service, 'technical rationality', and managerialism. As a result of a plethora of policy documents (including *Transforming Youth Work* (DfES, 2002), *Every Child Matters* (DfES, 2004), *Youth Matters* (DfES, 2005) and *Aiming High* (DCSF, 2007)), the management of youth work has undergone a profound shift. This chapter will examine this in the light of neoliberal principles.

### From social democracy to neoliberalism

The post-war period has been shaped by two major political and economic ideologies, which form two epochs which have been described as 'Welfarism' (1949–79) and 'Post-Welfarism' (1979–) (Clarke et al., 2000). Broadly speaking, the period of Welfarism can be seen to have been characterized by a commitment to social democracy, the period of Post-Welfarism by a commitment to neoliberalism.

The Depression of the 1920s and 1930s and the devastation of the Second World War had strengthened resolve for the creation of a better and more equal society. This was epitomized by the Beveridge Report, published in 1942, which identified five 'Giant Evils' in society: squalor, ignorance, want, idleness and disease, and went on to propose widespread reform to the system of social welfare in the UK, paving the way for the expansion of national insurance, the creation of the NHS and the arrival of what is popularly known as the welfare state. Keynesianism, the economic model that underpinned social democracy, advocated a mixed economy – predominantly private-sector but with government playing a prominent role which included interventionist policies.[1] The terms 'embedded liberalism' and 'social democratic consensus' have been used in reference to this period to indicate the ways in which 'market processes and entrepreneurial and corporate activities were surrounded by a web of social and political constraints and a regulatory environment that sometimes restrained ... economic and industrial activity' (Harvey, 2005: 11).

The period from the end of the Second World War to the early 1970s is generally regarded to have been a progressive era, referred to as the post-war 'Golden Age of Capitalism' (Marglin and Schor, 1992). The foundations of a number of the 'caring' or 'social' professions, including community work, social work and youth work, were put in place during this period (Davies, 1999a). In relation to youth work the government-commissioned Albemarle Report (ME, 1960) was seminal in this process and is credited with among other things the significant expansion of full-time youth workers, increased central and local government funding, and the raising of the status of youth work with the establishment of the Joint Negotiations Committee which set terms and conditions for youth workers at the national level, as well as the large-scale building programme for youth and community centres (Smith, 1997; Davies, 1999a). According to Mizen (2004), during this period youth became one of the biggest beneficiaries of the Keynesian strategy. He argues:

> Through criteria of age, more young people were brought within new and extended opportunities for schooling and expanded tertiary education free at the point of demand. The political commitment to full employment underwrote jobs for all school leavers and rising youth wages. The conditions under which youth crime and delinquency were regarded underwent a redefinition in terms of the needs of young offenders. And the young also found themselves incorporated into mainstream civil life through an expanded framework of civil, legal and political rights.
>
> (2004: 17)

In the early 1970s in an increasingly turbulent economic climate, the post-war social democratic consensus began to break down, prompting fundamental assumptions about the role of the state in the provision of social welfare to be questioned (Fraser, 2003). In the post-war years, despite the ideological differences between the right and left about the relative merits of capitalism and socialism and the role of the state in managing the economy, the consensus on welfare had been maintained. Now in the face of a global economic crisis right-wing voices of dissent began to dominate and an alternative neoliberal narrative emerged about how the economy should be managed and welfare delivered. From the 1980s onwards with the election of Margaret Thatcher in the UK in 1979 and Ronald Reagan in the United States in 1980, neoliberalism advanced as the dominant global economic and political ideology, based primarily upon a belief in the pre-eminent role of the market in maximizing human well-being.

According to Harvey, neoliberalism represents:

> A theory of political economic practices that proposes that human well-being can be best advanced by liberating individual entrepreneurial freedom characterised by strong private property rights, free markets and free trade. The role of the state is to create and preserve an institutional framework appropriate to such activities.
>
> (2005: 2)

Harvey's perspective on the role of the state underscores the point made earlier that whilst the excesses of the more strident form of neoliberalism promoted by the Conservatives were curbed somewhat by New Labour, the institutional framework and fundamentals remained in place and were actively promoted by the state, beyond the 1997 election.

## Neoliberalism, New Labour and managerialism

There is a tendency in much of the literature about management for it to be viewed in neutral, common sense terms in which 'technical expertise is privileged and decisions proceed through a rational process little impacted by the political world' (Skelcher et al., 2005: 586). However, management we would argue must be understood within its political context, and in this case neoliberalism's drive for change in public services and the delivery of welfare. But to understand the impact of neoliberalism on the management of youth and community work it is important to understand this broader institutional context and the technologies which have shaped and driven such changes. Citing the work of Clarke and Newman (1997), MacKinnon argues that:

> The local state has been restructured through the deployment of 'managerial technologies' designed to realise the objectives of neoliberal programmes of government. As a distinctive set of technologies and practices, managerialism can be seen as a product of the intersection of neoliberal political rationalities and business management prescriptions for organizational change to meet the competitive challenge of a global economy.
>
> (2000: 297)

Within this chapter we will examine two of these key neoliberal political rationalities and 'managerial' technologies – first, the introduction of private sector management practices into the public sector, often referred to as managerialism or New Public Management (NPM), and second, 'marketization': the introduction of competition which includes the shift in recent years to the contracting of services through a commissioning framework.

One of the core assumptions of neoliberalism has been a view that the state's management of public services has been inefficient and ineffective, and that the solution to this is the introduction of private sector management practices. What emerged was a move away from an incrementalist and particularistic style of management in favour of an economic, rationalist and generic model, based upon increasing importance paid to the 'three Es' of economy, efficiency and effectiveness (Farnham and Horton, 1996). Managerialism, or New Public Management as it became known, constituted a central feature of New Right policy driven forward by the Thatcher government in the 1980s and continued under successive New Labour governments. Managerialism is characterized by the assessment of 'quality' using external, objective benchmarks involving quantitative methods such as performance indicators and externally imposed targets (Clarke and Newman, 1997). Ball argues that this results in a combination of 'the terrors of performance and efficiency – performativity' (Ball 1998: 191). These have led directly to new forms of organizational control (Clarke, 1998: 176), which in turn undermines the level of trust placed on the professional (O'Neill 2002). Allied to this is a move from a more democratic managerial relationship to an autocratic one which

Clarke (1998) rightly describes as an assumption of the 'right to manage' in the pursuit of greater efficiency.

Before looking in more detail at the impact of neoliberalism and managerialism on youth work under New Labour, it is worth pausing, as there may be some who object to such comparisons between neoliberal Thatcherite policies and those of New Labour's 'Third Way'. We do, however, concur with Garrett's assertion that: 'any trace of progressive elements detectable in the endeavour to "transform" Children's Services [by New Labour] has been located within a neoliberal framework which is likely to constrain, nullify, or at best render ephemeral the more potentially positive components' (2009: 1). In a detailed critique highlighting the largely negative impact that neoliberalism has had on the so-called 'transformation' of children's services, Garrett makes a number of important points related to the ways in which the promoters of the transformation agenda have, in his terms, '*put language to work*' (Garrett, 2009: 3).

The first is that the 'change' agenda has been characterized by what he refers to as 'shallowness, depthlessness and superficiality' which can be related to 'the use of populist, frequently emotive slogans which are incessantly deployed in order to "brand" and "market" particular initiatives and to blur, or render porous, the distinction between the public and private sectors' (ibid.). Thus, according to Garrett, the 'Every Child Matters' and 'Sure Start' slogans, which mirrored developments in the United States with the 'No Child Left Behind' and 'Head Start' programmes, represented a 'branding of particular programmes of governance' which sought 'to mask the deeply ideological content of much of the "transformational reform agenda"' (ibid.).

Second, quoting Hall (2003), Garrett points to the complex and interwoven discourses which in combining the language of social democratic and neoliberal values has had the effect of deflecting the charge of neoliberalism away from the New Labour project. As Hall argues,

> New Labour is confusing … It combines economic liberalism with a commitment to 'active government'. More significantly, its grim alignment with the broad interest and values of corporate capital and power – the neoliberal, which is the *leading position* in its political repertoire – is paralleled by another *subaltern* programme, of a more social-democratic kind, running alongside. This is what people invoke when they insist defensively that New Labour, is not, after all, 'neoliberal'. The fact is that New Labour is a hybrid regime, composed of two strands. However, one strand – the neoliberal – is the dominant position. The other strand – the social democratic – is subordinate.
>
> (2003: 19)

The clearest example of the primacy of neoliberal values at the heart of New Labour's reforms of youth work was the thankfully failed attempt to 'marketize' youth work. At the heart of the Youth Matters (DfES, 2005) reform agenda was an attempt via the introduction of the 'Opportunity Card' to introduce a market in the provision of youth work. The idea was to give each young person in the country a 'debit' card which would enable young people to be direct purchasers of provision. The government proposed that the cards would provide discount on a range of things to do and places to go and could also be topped up by parents and young people (DfES, 2005: 5). In addition the government would also top up the opportunity cards of disadvantaged

13–16-year-olds. This subsidy would be withheld from young people engaging in unacceptable and anti-social behaviour and the cards suspended or withdrawn (ibid.).

It has been noted that this reframing of young people as consumers runs totally counter to the notion of civil society out of which youth work had developed (Jeffs and Smith, 2006). Also by ensuring that youth work providers were in direct competition, this policy 'threatened to "drive a coach and horses" through the network of youth projects' (Ord, 2007: 107). However, one should not be overly surprised at this mismatch between New Labour's apparent commitment to meeting the needs of young people and what for some was a throwback to Thatcher; as Hall (2003) argues, despite appearances it is ultimately the neoliberal thread which dominates New Labour's ideology. The hybrid character is not simply a static formation, however: it is the *process* which combines the two elements which matters. The process is 'transformist'. The latter always remains subordinate to and dependent on the former, and *is constantly being 'transformed' into* the former dominant one (2003: 19).

Third, for Garrett, is the important way in which language has been deployed under neoliberalism in general. Garrett urges those situated within children's services and the institutions governing entry into the 'caring' professions 'to think more deeply and more politically ... of how power relations operate through language ... and ... of how key words and phrases can continually – but often imperceptibly – contribute to the solidifying of neoliberal hegemonic order' (2009: 26). 'Partnership' and 'empowerment' are examples of two such words, often bandied around, not least within the youth and community work field. As has been argued in relation to community development, such words have been co-opted under neoliberalism (Bunyan, 2010) to reflect the upbeat rhetoric of neoliberal programmes of change and to emphasize depoliticized consensus-based versions over and against alternative adversarial-based forms of change.

## Neoliberalism and youth work policy

Despite claims that the Thatcherite era was having a detrimental effect on youth work practice, for example Jeffs and Smith's claim that the emergence of a focus on the control and surveillance of groups of young people, such as the young, offenders, homeless, or unemployed, indicated 'a drift towards a new authoritarianism' (1994: 28), to a large extent youth work escaped direct policy intervention during the eighteen years of Thatcherite governments, and suffered from neglect (Davies, 1999b: 13). Whether deemed too insignificant to bother with, indicated perhaps by the derision which was displayed to the only government-commissioned report on youth work (the Thompson Report, DES 1982) during that period (Davies, 1999b) or whether there were 'bigger fish to fry' and the focus was on the large institutions of education, social services and the NHS, either way it was not until the arrival of New Labour that youth work experienced directly the impact of neoliberal managerial reforms.

Within its first year, the New Labour administration had commissioned a report on the youth service, entitled *England's Youth Service: The 1998 Audit* (NYA/DfEE, 1998). It claimed to be the most comprehensive review and audit of youth services to date; but it is noteworthy that this was primarily concerned with financial auditing and an assessment of the varying costs of youth work. But it was also concerned with the quality of the work: 'A notable feature of this report is the variability in youth provision across the country' (1998: 3), clearly implying that some was good but much was poor. It is unfortunate that the context of eighteen years of successive cuts to local government youth services under the previous Conservative government (Davies 1999b) was not used to explain this alleged poor quality. However, the report was clearly being utilized to justify the need for reform. This was heralded shortly after by the first 'Transforming Youth Work' policy document entitled *Developing Youth Work for Young People* (DfEE, 2001).

Youth workers could take some solace from a repositioning of youth work and some recognition from government about its role and significance. The report acknowledged that: 'Young People need good quality advice, guidance, support and personal development opportunities to help make the transition to adult and working life' (DfEE, 2001: 5) and more importantly: 'the youth service will be the source of expertise and champions of youth work and personal development, both as a service in its own right and as a contributor to the Connexions service' (DfEE, 2001: 8). This policy coincided with the launch of the Connexions service and raised concerns amongst workers that youth work would be subsumed within it (Davies, 2008). More pressing concerns were raised with the claim in the document that the youth service needed to improve significantly: 'the quality being achieved is at best variable with slightly more than one in three unsatisfactory and providing poor value for money' (DfEE, 2001: 8). The major reforms of youth work practice, and the subsequent management of it, were soon to arrive with the publication of *Transforming Youth Work: Resourcing Excellent Youth Services* (DfES, 2002).

This document, like many New Labour policies, again puts 'words to work' (Garrett, 2009: 3). At face value there is much that can be used to signify a positive outlook: a description of youth work values,[2] a pledge to young people which included commitment to 'a safe, warm well-equipped meeting place within reasonable distance of home' (DfES, 2002: 22), as well as a recommendation, but sadly not an assurance, of a minimum expenditure level for youth work of £100 per head. However, the real issue at the heart of transforming youth work was an introduction of externally imposed targets on youth work practice. Indeed, these targets are one of the lasting legacies of *Transforming Youth Work* because they were incorporated directly into the best value performance indicators that all local authorities would need to report against. Thus the BVPI 221a, 221b, what youth workers know as the 'accreditation' and 'recorded outcome' targets would have a real and significant impact on the delivery of youth work and its subsequent management[3] (see Chapter 9 for an examination of the impact of targets).

This shift in youth work to objective-driven performance targets is directly attributable to the new managerial practices which emerged from the 1980s onwards. According to Smith, *Transforming Youth Work* is 'clothed in the rhetoric of new managerialism'. He comments:

> The concerns and direction of Transforming Youth Work are clear here. Using a business model, they want youth work that is targeted, concerned with meeting ('delivering') Connexions requirements (keeping young people in touch with the labour market and continuing education), and that is outcome-focused ... The rhetoric of managerialism has bitten so deep that it has contributed significantly to the subversion of distinctive purposes, conditions and tasks.

(2001)

Another important feature of the Transforming Youth Work agenda was the importance placed on the external inspection regime of Ofsted. In 2001 the revised Ofsted inspections framework was published, and this was to play a significant role in providing an external system of monitoring and evaluation of services against these externally imposed benchmarks (DfES, 2002). Indeed, it also was proposed that the DfES would as a result of consistent failure to achieve satisfactory inspections have the power to: 'outsource the service beyond direct local authority delivery' (DfES, 2002: 28). Thus the ground was prepared for the possibilities of more diverse forms of delivery consistent with neoliberal ideology based upon the introduction of competition and a commissioning framework for the design and delivery of youth work.

## Partnership, commissioning and competition

While partnership is nothing new, in that youth work organizations have always worked together to a greater or lesser extent, under New Labour it has taken on a pivotal role (Taylor and Warburton, 2003). The election of New Labour, after almost two decades of Conservative rule, was greeted with widespread approval by the voluntary and community sector and the sense of a new dawn was cemented by the institution of the 'social compact', an agreement between government and the third sector which formally acknowledged the right of the sector 'to campaign, to comment on Government policy and to challenge that policy irrespective of any funding relationship that might exist' (Home Office, 1998: para. 9:1).

The emphasis upon partnership is exemplified by the use of the term 'joined up government' by Tony Blair, when he launched the Social Exclusion Unit in 1997, claiming that: 'Pressing problems facing government, such as social exclusion, crime, environment, family and competitiveness, do not fit neatly into departmental boundaries' (Mulgan, 2005: 175). However, partnership exemplifies what Hall (2003) referred to as the hybrid nature of New Labour policy and much of the discourse on partnership reflects the progressive 'social democratic' strand. This includes the democratizing of the policy process which is characterized by a shift from government to governance and the opening up of 'new spaces' and opportunities for actors who in the past had been excluded from the policy process (Geddes, 2006). It also places an emphasis on the involvement of service users and communities (Tett, 2005), as well as on networking and the building of inter-organizational relationships (Somers and Bradford, 2006).

During the thirteen years of New Labour, through which policy on partnership has developed, the 'leading strand', and dominant position, of neoliberalism, as Hall (2003) suggested, comes to the fore. Whilst initially there seemed to be an emphasis on cooperation (Taylor, 1997), it is evident that ultimately it is competition and an emphasis on 'the market' which takes precedence. As well as of course the centrality of the three E's (efficiency, effectiveness and economy), as Morse and McNamara (2006) argue, striving for better and more efficient use of scarce resources is never very far from partnership policy and practice. Confirmation of this can be found in the importance placed on commissioning within New Labour policy (DfES, 2003; DfES, 2005; DCSF, 2007).

Sercombe notes this shift in policy and how this has affected the voluntary sector in particular, and how historically:

Government funding was mainly in the form of grants to community organizations to support services, proposed and initiated by the community. Often services are now designed and initiated by governments and put out for tender on a payment for service basis. Agencies are now effectively agents of government, still with some scope for autonomous action, but within increasingly prescribed limits.

(2010: 56)

As a result of the establishment of Children's Trusts, local authorities are now considered in many cases not as 'deliverers' of youth services but as 'enablers' commissioning the services from a variety of public, private and third sector organizations. Thus providers are now in competition with each other to secure the necessary financial resources with which to deliver youth work (Davies and Merton, 2009).

The example of Northamptonshire illustrates the worst aspects of neoliberal policy, how the establishment of a market is used to both undermine existing provision as well as substantially reduce public expenditure, whilst at the same time putting 'words to work' (Garrett, 2009) to provide the impression of an overwhelming success. Northamptonshire County Council defines youth service commissioning as:

The process by which a local authority identifies the needs of its population of young people, and plans, and delivers services for them, from within its own resources or from a range of providers in the voluntary sector, district council and independent sectors.

(Northamptonshire, 2006)

However, the process of commissioning of the youth service started from the premise that it: 'proposed to reduce Youth Service funding by £2.5m (from £3.8m to £1.3m)' (ibid.).

Thus over a two-year period, Northamptonshire County Council managed to achieve significant reductions in expenditure whilst at the same time claiming:

Young people in Northamptonshire have benefited from the council's decision to commission youth services ... Commissioning services rather than providing them directly was seen as the best way for Northamptonshire County Council to achieve its aim of becoming a smaller, more enabling authority. It enabled the council to improve its services in order to achieve better outcomes for children, young people and families, and use the resources available to do this as efficiently as possible.

(LGA, 2008)

Despite wholesale cuts in funding the narrative is one of unqualified success as the council becomes more 'enabling' and partnership-focused. Beneath the gloss, however, the reality is that whilst the burden of responsibility has shifted to the voluntary and community sector (often, it should be said, welcomed by some sections of the sector), it has taken place within a reduced budgetary framework and an ever tighter and increasingly constrained target and outcome-focused straitjacket. In the process the structure of the voluntary and community sector has been fundamentally reshaped, with many of the larger organizations effectively becoming quasi-governmental in nature and the independence and adversarial role of the sector being significantly eroded. (For further exploration of the impact of the current climate on the voluntary sector, see Chapter 13.)

## Conclusion

Youth work and the way it is managed has fundamentally changed as a result of the neoliberal policy context, which although introduced under Thatcher, had considerably more impact under New Labour. A central theme in this chapter has been the focus on neoliberal discourse and the ways in which language has been 'put to work' by successive governments to 'solidify the neoliberal hegemonic order' (Garrett, 2009: 26). As a result both youth work delivery and its subsequent management has undergone a fundamental shift with the implementation of managerialist practices, target setting and competition now at the heart of youth work practice.

In the aftermath of New Labour's defeat and the election of the coalition government, whilst the emphasis has changed towards the 'shrinking of the state' and growth of the 'big society', the underlying discourse is likely to remain the same. There is little sign of a turning away from neoliberalism and its underlying tenets and values. On the contrary, in an increasingly hostile economic climate it is likely that many of the key features of neoliberalism, including a preference for 'private' over 'public' sector, economic stringency and the allocation of resources through a competitive contract framework, will remain firmly in place. This will present significant challenges to the youth work sector as a whole, and to the way it is managed. If there is to be any form of meaningful resistance, or engagement, with the dominant neoliberal hegemonic order, then youth workers, those who manage youth work, as well as the institutions that provide training and education, will need to think more deeply, and politically, about the wider context of youth work, and how it is managed.

## Questions for reflection and discussion

1   Can you identify examples of how the neoliberal values of individualism and competition are impacting upon the management of youth work?
2   To what extent has the profession of youth and community work uncritically adopted the language of neoliberalism?
3   What has been the impact on youth work as a result of New Labour's policies on the management of youth work?
4   To what extent, and by what means, can the dominant values of neoliberalism be countered through alternative managerial practices?

## Notes

1 Interestingly, in the wake of the global economic crisis in recent years, there has been a resurgence of interest in Keynesian economics and strategy and government intervention into the most fundamental of neoliberal markets: the finance and banking sector.
2 Many of those listed had appeared previously in articles by Bernard Davies which the DfES failed to acknowledge.
3 Although the BVPIs were formally removed in 2009 as reporting measures, their acceptance by managers as key mechanisms for evidencing 'quality' ensures that they are likely to remain (Davies and Merton, 2009).

## Further reading

Davies, B. (2008) *The New Labour Years: A History of the Youth Service in England, Volume 3*, Leicester: Youth Work Press.

Garrett, P. M. (2009) *'Transforming' Children's Services? Social Work, Neoliberalism and the 'Modern' World*, Maidenhead: McGraw-Hill Education/Open University Press.

Harvey, D. (2005) *A Brief History of Neoliberalism*, Oxford: Oxford University Press.

Sandel, M. (2010) 'Markets and morals: a new citizenship', Reith Lectures, available at downloads.bbc.co.uk/.../20090609_thereithlectures_marketsandmorals.rtf (accessed 4 April 2011).

## References

Ball, S. J. (1998) 'Performativity and fragmentation in post modern schooling', in J. Carter (ed.) *Post-Modernity and the Fragmentation of Welfare*, London: Routledge, pp. 187–203.

Bunyan, P. (2010) 'Broad-based organizing in the UK: reasserting the centrality of political activity in community development', *Community Development Journal*, 45(1): 111–27. Oxford: Oxford University Press and Community Development Journal.

Clarke, J. (1998) 'Thriving on chaos? Managerialism and social welfare', in J. Carter (ed.) *Post-Modernity and the Fragmentation of Welfare*, London: Routledge, pp. 171–186.

Clarke, J., Gewirtz, S. and McClaughlin, E. (eds) (2000) *New Managerialism, New Welfare*, London: Sage/Open University Press.

Clarke, J. and Newman, J. E. (1997) *The Managerial State: Power, Politics and Ideology in the Remaking of Social Welfare*, London: Sage.

Davies, B. (1999a) *From Voluntaryism to Welfare State: A History of the Youth Service in England, Volume 1*, Leicester: Youth Work Press.

——(1999b) *The Thatcher Years: A History of the Youth Service in England, Volume 2*, Leicester: Youth Work Press.

——(2008) *The New Labour Years: A History of the Youth Service in England, Volume 3*, Leicester: Youth Work Press.

Davies, B. and Merton, B. (2009) *Squaring the Circle*, Leicester: De Montfort University. Available at www.dmu.ac.uk/Images/Squaring%20the%20Circle_tcm6–50166.pdf

DCSF (2007) *Aiming High for Young People: A Ten Year Strategy for Positive Activities*, London: Department for Children, Schools and Families.

DES (1982) *Experience and Participation. Review Group on the Youth Service in England* ('The Thompson Report'), London: Department of Education and Science.

DfEE (2001) *Developing Youth Work for Young People*, London: Department for Education and Employment.

DfES (2001) *Transforming Youth Work: Developing Youth Work for Young People*, London: Department for Education and Skills.

——(2002) *Transforming Youth Work: Resourcing Excellent Youth Services*, London: Department for Education and Skills.

——(2003) *Every Child Matters*, London: Department for Education and Skills.

——(2004) *Every Child Matters: Change for Children*, London: Department for Education and Skills.

——(2005) *Youth Matters*, London: Department for Education and Skills.

Farnham, D. and Horton, S. (eds) (1996) *Managing the New Public Services* (2nd edn) London: Macmillan.

Fraser, D. (2003) *The Evolution of the British Welfare State*, Basingstoke: Palgrave Macmillan.

Garrett, P.M. (2009) *'Transforming' Children's Services? Social Work, Neoliberalism and the 'Modern' World*, Maidenhead: McGraw-Hill Education/Open University Press.

Geddes, M. (2006) 'Partnership and the limits to local governance in England: institutionalist analysis and neoliberalism', *International Journal of Urban and Regional Research*, 30(1): 76–97.

Hall, S. (2003) 'New Labour's double-shuffle', *Soundings*, 24: 10–25.

Harvey, D. (2005) *A Brief History of Neoliberalism*, Oxford: Oxford University Press.

Home Office (1998) *Compact on Relations between Government and the Voluntary and Community Sector in England*, London: Home Office.

Jeffs, T. and Smith, M. K. (1994) 'Young people, youth work and a new authoritarianism', *Youth and Policy*, no. 46 (Autumn): 17–32.

——'Where is *Youth Matters* taking us?' *Youth and Policy*, no. 91 (Spring): 23–39.

LGA (Local Government Association) (2008) 'Commissioning Services' (Online). Available at www.lga.gov.uk/lga/core/page.do?pageId=1251611 (Accessed 2 April 2010).

MacKinnon, D. (2000) 'Managerialism, governmentality and the state: a neo-Foucauldian approach to local economic governance', *Political Geography*, 19(3): 293–314.

Marglin, S. and Schor, J. (eds) (1992) *The Golden Age of Capitalism: Reinterpreting the Postwar Experience*, New York: Oxford University Press.

ME (1960) *Youth Service in England and Wales* (Albemarle Report). London: Ministry of Education, HMSO.

Mizen, P. (2004) *The Changing State of Youth*, Basingstoke: Palgrave Macmillan.

Morse, S. and McNamara, N. (2006) 'Analysing institutional partnerships in development: a contract between equals or a loaded process?' *Progress in Development Studies*, 6(4): 321–36.

Mulgan, G. (2005) 'Joined up government: past, present, future', in V. Bogdanor (ed.) *Joined Up Government*, Oxford: Oxford University Press, pp. 175–87.

Northamptonshire County Council Cabinet (2006) *Youth Service: The Transition from a Direct Delivery Service to an Enabling Service through a Commissioning Strategy*. Report by the Director for Children and Young People, 19 June.

NYA/DfEE (1998) *England's Youth Service: The 1998 Audit*, Leicester: NYA.

O'Neill, O. (2002) *A Question of Trust: The BBC Reith Lectures, 2002*, Cambridge: Cambridge University Press.

Ord, J. (2007) *Youth Work Process Product and Practice: Creating an Authentic Curriculum in Work with Young People*, Lyme Regis: RHP.

Sercombe, H. (2010) *Youth Work Ethics*, London: Sage.

Skelcher, C., Mathur, N. and Smith, M. (2005) 'The public governance of collaborative spaces: discourse, design and democracy', *Public Administration*, 83(3): 573–96.

Smith, D. S. (1997) 'The eternal triangle: youth work, the youth problem and social policy', in I. Ledgerwood and N. Kendra (eds) *The Challenge of the Future. Towards the New Millennium for the Youth Service*, Lyme Regis: Russell House, pp. 21–40.

Smith, M. K. (2001) 'Transforming youth work', *The Encyclopaedia of Informal Education*, www.infed.org/youthwork/transforming.htm (accessed 25 March 2010).

Smith, M. K. and Doyle, M. E. (2002) 'The Albemarle Report and the development of youth work in England and Wales', *The Encyclopaedia of Informal Education*, www.infed.org/youthwork/albemarle_report.htm

Somers, J. and Bradford, S. (2006) 'Discourses of partnership in multi-agency working in the community and voluntary sectors in Ireland', *Irish Journal of Sociology*, 15(2): 67–85.

Taylor, M. (1997) *The Best of Both Worlds: The Voluntary Sector and Local Government*, York: Joseph Rowntree Foundation.

Taylor, M. and Warburton, D. (2003) 'Legitimacy and the role of UK third sector organisations in the policy process', *Voluntas: International Journal of Voluntary and Non-profit Organisations*, 14(3): 321–328.

Tett, L. (2005) 'Partnerships, community groups and social inclusion', *Studies in Continuing Education*, 27(1): 1–15.

# 3 'Theories' of youth work management

## Roger Harrison and Jon Ord

For many, perhaps a majority of youth work managers, their careers began as face-to-face workers, with management responsibilities being acquired as a necessary but not always welcome part of progression up the career ladder. However, in the main these responsibilities are acquired with little formal training or education on the 'theory' of management, beyond what they may have studied many years previously on a qualifying course (Bracy, 2007). As with all fields of practice, the theory which is applicable to managing in a youth work context is by no means stable or settled, but continually subject to change and controversy. At a time when strengthening leadership and management has become increasingly utilized as a strategy for raising standards in public services, including youth work (DfES 2002; DfCSF, 2007), it is important for practitioners to maintain a critical awareness of the ideas and assumptions which underpin these strategies so that they can make informed decisions about appropriate management practices rather than responding to the whim of the dominant management discourse.

This chapter aims to do two things: first to outline the main theoretical approaches which underpin current discourses of management in youth work, providing the language through which we attempt to understand and explain management practices; and second to take a step back from these explanations and to ask more fundamental questions about the position and role which management has achieved in recent times, and what effects this has had on current practices of youth work.

## Theoretical approaches to management

It is widely accepted that there are four theoretical approaches which underpin management, they are listed below in order of their historical emergence.

| | |
|---|---|
| Classic or scientific theory of management | (circa 1910) |
| Humanistic theory | (circa 1950) |
| Systems theory | (circa 1980) |
| Contingency theory | (circa 2000) |

(Cole, 2004; Mullins, 2007; Hannagan, 2008)

### *Classic or scientific theory*

Classic or scientific theory of management has its origins in early industrialization and in the development of production lines. Importantly it is founded in a belief that management is rational and principles can be developed to organize productivity and increase efficiency, hence the notion of 'scientific' management (Cole, 2004). It was originally concerned with routine manufacturing, and the organization of the tasks required to produce specific goods. Importantly, management is seen as objective and impersonal. The original 'experiment' in scientific management was performed by Taylor at the turn of the twentieth century (Taylor, 1947). He analysed the practices of the men shovelling coal at the Bethlehem steel works, with particular attention focused on the measurement and specification of activities of production. He made a careful examination of all organizational tasks, standardizing many tasks and procedures, and introducing systems of reward and punishment. 'The results were impressive: the work of 400–600 men was being done by 140' (Cole, 2004: 19).

It is easy to think that such practices have little relevance to the world of youth work. However, the effects of what is often known as 'Taylorism' are profound and far-reaching. Whilst few managers would see themselves as 'scientific' in their approach, many are however convinced that it is possible to find the 'one best way' of doing things (Gilbreth, cited in Cole, 2004: 19). And the remnants of scientific theory remain in such concepts as 'time and motion'. Youth workers are increasingly asked to account for their time in a 'Taylorist' manner. It is not unheard of for a youth worker's week to be broken down into 15-minute intervals, each of which needs to be accounted for specifically in terms of productivity and output. Such 'quantifiable' measures of performance independent of the people, or their varying needs, are indicative of a classic or scientific approach.

Evidence of scientism appears in such concepts as performance-related pay, with its incorporation of incentives, which though rare, is appearing in youth work organizations. The influence of the classic or scientific approach is more commonly found in more mundane management practices such as the insistence on specific ratios of workers to young people, in youth work settings independent of the 'qualities' of the staff involved. It could be argued that two high quality, experienced youth workers who have good relationships with the young people in the project, are far better than three, four or even more workers who are neither experienced, nor have good relationships. It could even be argued that one very good worker would be better than three or four inexperienced ones, but the adherence to ratios is often adhered to strictly. Another example of this approach would be the increasing emergence of guidance documents, policies, and procedures governing the practice of youth work, from induction, staff development, and health and safety, as well as more established practices such as street-based youth work. It could be argued that the responsiveness of the individual practitioner 'enabled' to take account of the vagaries of the particular setting that they practice in is being undermined by such regimentation and routinization, all of which originates from a classic or scientific theoretical position.

Clearly there is a need for consistency of approach in certain circumstances, and in some ways classic or scientific management does enable a degree of equity and fairness and allows for the efficient organization of tasks. However, at its worst classic or scientific theory has an exclusive focus on the task, independent of the people performing the task and/or the unique environment and circumstances in which the task takes place. Management in these circumstances is reduced to Fayol's original definition: 'to plan, to organize, to command, to coordinate and to control' (Fayol, 1916, cited in Cole, 2004: 16). As Mullins suggests, management in this sense conceives of 'organizations without people' (Mullins 2007: 54).

### Humanist theory

The humanist theory is arguably more important in youth work management, but increasingly less common in the current managerialist climate. This approach to management was a response to the mechanistic and impersonal approaches of the classic/ scientific perspective. It developed out of theories of social and developmental psychology of the 1950s and it argues there is too much focus on the 'task', and not enough on the people involved. A definition from that period characterizes the specific shift in focus, depicting management as: 'a *social* process, for planning and regulating the operations of the enterprise towards some agreed objective' (Brech, 1957, cited in Cole, 2004: 24). The key issue for a humanist manager is 'motivation' and attention to the needs of employees. It is no surprise that the 1950s also saw the emergence of Maslow's popular hierarchy of needs (Maslow, 1954). Within this new approach employees were not simply 'wage slaves' motivated exclusively by reward and punishment, but complex human beings who had a variety of their needs met through their work. Even an application of the simplistic hierarchy provided by Maslow begins to show that employees could be equally motivated by the social relationships that are formed at work or the esteem which they feel as a result of the position they are in, as much as the wages they receive.

Interestingly, the origins of humanist theory lie in a study which still has relevance to the management of youth work. Known as the Hawthorne studies, conducted by Elton Mayo in the 1930s, they were an attempt to improve productivity by altering lighting levels in an assembly room; researchers were at first baffled by the fact that regardless of what alterations were made, improvements in productivity were achieved. They concluded that it was simply the fact that attention was being paid to the workers that produced the greater productivity. This became known as the Hawthorne effect. Latterly this work was developed by Parker Follett (1940), Maslow (1954), and Likert (1961), each of whom attempted to assess the importance of 'social and belonging needs, as opposed to the needs of the task' (Cole, 2004: 35). Workers were no longer thought of as the rational and economic beings – 'like components or cogs in a machine' – previously assumed by classical theorists. Instead individuals were now thought of as having a variety of complex needs which were met through their work. They concluded that social interaction is of fundamental importance, and people work well if they feel valued. As a result, notions of 'good management' have become linked with the achievement of workers' individual potential through increased levels of autonomy and responsibility. It is important in the current managerialist climate, to remember that studies by Mintzberg (1973) and Kotter (1996) found successful managers spend little time analysing tasks; instead they cultivate networks and personal contacts.

Humanist theory is perhaps most evident in the formal practices of staff development, appraisal, and supervision. Each of which, in theory at least, should take note of, and respond to the 'needs' of the workers. (The issue of supervision and worker's needs is explored more fully in Chapter 8.) Youth work managers should perhaps remember that most youth workers are highly motivated to do their job, many regarding it as a vocation or a calling (Doyle, 1999). Managers must therefore appreciate what motivates workers if they are to successfully manage them. Youth work is also a value-laden profession (Banks, 2010; Young, 2005; Jeffs and Smith, 2005) and therefore youth workers' managers need to engage with, and understand the values that underpin the work youth workers do. This is an issue which is no doubt exacerbated by the context of integrated services, where youth workers may be managed by someone who does not have a youth work background.

The humanist theory is, however, not without its criticisms; for example, Schein (1965) argued in his characterization of 'complex man' that no single management style can succeed in improving the performance of all workers. It should be acknowledged that the motives of an individual may be extremely complex, and liable to change over time. And perhaps more importantly, a high level of satisfaction does not necessarily lead to increased productivity. That is if a worker is motivated by a particular need, for example achievement or recognition, and that need is met, their motivation may well reduce.

The two schools of classic/scientific and humanist portray opposing but not mutually exclusive approaches to management, and it is argued that it is good practice in management to focus on both the achievement of specific tasks, as well as attending to the motivational needs of workers. Hannagan (2008) plots these two factors on a graph and concludes that good management needs to successfully incorporate both approaches, referring to this as 'team management'. He argues poor management results from too much focus exclusively on the task, leading to what he calls 'authoritarian management'. Hannagan sees equally poor management resulting from too much focus on the needs of employees, describing this as 'country club management', characterized as an organization where everyone feels acknowledged and their needs accommodated but where there is a lack of focus on the task in hand. Importantly in the current climate, questions could be asked as to whether each of the two traditional schools of management are given equal priority. Given Clarke's (1998) emphasis on new managerialism's *'right to manage'* it is likely that *'the command and control'* of classic/scientific management theory is given priority.

### Systems theory

Systems theory 'in principle' accords with Hannagan's (2008) demand for an equal focus on both task and person. It was an attempt to incorporate the positive aspects of each of the two previous opposing theoretical positions. More importantly, it was an attempt to conceptualize the whole organization and its interrelated parts, as well as an appreciation of the 'continual interaction with the broader external environment of which it is a part' (Mullins, 2007: 55). Systems theory enables theorists to see management not just in terms of the task or the people but as multi-dimensional, and it attempts to explain how the people, the structure, technology and the environment react together to enable the organization to achieve its objectives.

Ford et al. (2005) argue systems theory is the dominant perspective of management, claiming: 'Most organisations use an open systems model approach to understand and monitor their performance' (2005: 163). Ford et al. go on to suggest that this invariably 'involves identifying inputs, the process of transforming inputs into outputs, and the outcomes these can lead to' (2005: 163); see Figure 3.1 below.

The adoption of systems theory and the utilization of private sector practices emphasizing efficient and effective transformation of 'inputs' into 'outputs' in youth work management practice is a stark reminder of the impact of new managerialism. Whilst it may be the case that these practices have 'streamlined' some youth work organizations and enabled efficient use of resources in accordance with the third 'E' of

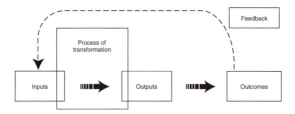

*Figure 3.1* Open systems management model (Ford et al., 2005: 163)

new managerialism: 'economy' (Farnham and Horton, 1993), importantly Mullins (2007) talks exclusively about business organizations when talking about the usefulness of systems theory. Questions need to be asked about the 'fit' between educational organizations and the input–output model. It has been argued that the educational 'process' cannot be reduced to a simplistic conversion of inputs and outputs (Ord, 2004; 2007) not least because of the incidental nature of outcomes in informal education (Smith, 1988). (This issue is explored in more detail in Chapter 6 in the discussion about planning.)

Systems theory has developed the theory of management beyond the dualistic notions of 'task' and 'person' and has attempted (at least in its fullest sense) to account for the complexity of management practices. However, where it is represented as a simplistic linear process of transforming inputs to outputs, it has been closely aligned with new managerialism's emphasis on efficiency and effectiveness, rather than with a serious attempt to understand and articulate the complexities and uniqueness of each organization and its relationship with its environment.

### *Contingency theory*

Contingency theory is premised on a rejection of classic/scientific theory's belief that there is one best form of management, and does not hold to the belief that generalizable principles can be established across organizations (Mullins, 2007). It is also, however, critical of human relations schools' denial of the importance of structure. Contingency theory can also be seen as a development of systems theory, in that it builds on the attempt by the systems approach to determine the most appropriate organizational design and management style for a given set of circumstances. The starting point for contingency theory is therefore an appreciation of the uniqueness of each organizational and management setting. As Mullins suggests:

> The contingency approach takes the view that there is no one best, universal structure. There are a large number of variables, or situational factors, which influence organizational design and performance. The contingency approach emphasises the need for flexibility.
>
> (Mullins, 2007: 603)

Importantly the 'success of the organization is dependent upon a range of situational variables' (Mullins, 2007: 41). The range of variables is considerable in the complex environment of modern (youth work) management. Although Handy (1999) tries to simplify these by suggesting that the three key variables managers have to grapple with are: 'people', 'work and structures' and 'systems and procedures'; and that these are set in the context of: 'the goals of the organization', 'the technology available', and 'the culture of the organization'. Another very popular method of identifying the key variables in a management and organizational setting is McKinsey's 7S model, which identified: strategy, structure, systems, style, staff, skills, and shared goals as the key variables (Mullins, 2007: 757).

Clearly, contingency theory offers a challenge to the traditional conceptualizations of management, in its rejection of generalizable principles, replacing them with a search for what 'best fits' the uniqueness of the organizational context. It also offers a challenge to the dominance of systems theory and an exclusive conceptualization of organizations in terms of a conversion of inputs to outputs, by arguing that the most appropriate management practices, structures and systems, etc., all need to be contingent on the unique circumstances of the setting within which they operate. Youth work management therefore needs to appreciate the unique and particular 'variables' operating within our educational practices. That means youth work management needs to take account of the differences between youth work and other forms of practice, as well as appreciate the differences within youth work itself, for example between detached work and centre-based youth work (see Chapters 9 and 10).

Whilst it is the case that each new theoretical position was created in response to identified weaknesses of the previous approach, each new approach did not supersede its predecessor. Elements of each position remain, with the potential to inform contemporary management practices. With the arrival of new managerialism in youth work, and an emphasis on 'the right to manage', it could be argued that the 'command and control' of previous classic/scientific approaches has again come to the fore. Indeed, Farnham and Horton suggest:

> The origins of the new managerialism have been attributed to New Right ideology ... but its roots lie further back in classical scientific management and the ideas of Frederick Taylor and Henri Fayol.
>
> (1993: 239)

In the context of youth work, systems theory is also clearly dominant (Ford et al., 2005). But it is argued that in the main it has been used for the ease with which organizations can be brought to account, rather than to comprehend the complexities of organizations, and articulate the management practices that are required by such complexities. It would be to their advantage for youth work managers to understand the range of theoretical approaches in order to have an informed understanding of management. As a result they would be in a better position to develop a set of appropriate management 'practices'. In addition, managers need to ensure that the important tenets of humanism – that productivity invariably increases when the motivations and needs of workers are taken into account – are not lost in the current 'climate of accountability'.

## A postmodern perspective on youth work management

So far this chapter has represented management theory as a rational project whose object is to gain clearer and more sophisticated understandings of how managers might conduct themselves to get the best out of their workforce. Whilst systems theory and contingency theory present more subtle and nuanced understandings of how organizations work than do classic or scientific approaches, they are nevertheless engaged in a similar project – to discover generalized descriptions of how organizations work and therefore how they might be managed more efficiently. This is at the heart a rationalist project aimed at controlling human activity through the development of knowledge. In this second part of the chapter we look at a perspective on management which raises different questions about the role of management theory.

One way of reading the development of management theory as we have described it in the previous section is as a progressive movement from simple mechanistic understandings of how organizations work to more sophisticated and contingent ones. We might describe this as a classic modernist narrative, one in which knowledge increases through scientific inquiry, leading to better, if more complex, models of how organizations work and how managers might therefore behave. Modernism can be thought of as a belief system which views the world as susceptible to rational explanation and human control. It is grounded in a positivist paradigm where meaning can be captured through empirical enquiry. It is through gaining knowledge that we can gain power and control over organizations and those who work within them. The building of knowledge and expertise about management provides a grand narrative of progress allowing greater efficiency and effectiveness through 'ordering social relations according to the model of functional rationality' (Cooper and Burrell, 1988: 96). In contrast, a postmodern perspective suggests meaning is mercurial, always negotiable and subject to change over time and between places. Rather than an object which can be pursued and eventually captured and described, what is real remains fluid and continually in the process of being constructed and reconstructed through language and human interaction. Meanings are 'made', that is, constituted through language at particular times and places, rather than 'found' as pre-existing entities.

From a postmodern perspective the question to ask is not 'what do we know about management?', but 'how has a discourse of management emerged and what are the effects on people and organizations of explanations based on this discourse?' Here attention shifts away from what is regarded as a futile pursuit of truth about management, with its seductive promises of best practice, improved performance and predictable outcomes, towards an examination of the processes through which the idea of management as a route to improving practices becomes accepted as 'common sense'.

> Discourse analysts are much more interested in studying the process of construction itself, how 'truths' emerge, how social realities and identities are built and the consequences of these, than working out what 'really happened'.
>
> (Wetherell, 2001: 16)

To illustrate this approach from other studies in the field of education, Edwards (2001) uses a form of discourse analysis to show how notions of individual learner needs construct characterizations of learners and require particular kinds of pedagogical responses. Nicholl and Harrison (2003) use a similar analysis of curriculum statements about teacher competence to show how discourses of 'good' and 'professional teaching' are constituted. Soreide (2007) analyses documents which specify the content of school curricula, which produce what she terms 'public narratives' which constitute what teaching is and 'how teachers should think about themselves as teachers'. In each case the focus is on the way in which knowledge and meaning are constructed through discourse, which Foucault refers to as 'identifiable collections of utterances ... which determine ... what may be said, by whom, in what context and with what effect' (Gordon, 1994: xvi).

From this perspective what is taken as 'real' is instead considered to be constituted through discourse. The discourse provides the means through which descriptions of the world are organized and presented in ways which make them appear credible and objective. The notion of discourse is helpful in raising awareness of the processes through which changes to our ways of thinking about the work we do with young people are mobilized and enacted. Foucault uses the idea of discourse to mean regimes of truth which powerfully influence the meanings we attach to contemporary developments. Their power depends on how far they are able to naturalize, to bestow a 'taken-for-granted' status on understandings which are historically and culturally located. As Foucault puts this:

> Each society has its own regime of truth, its 'general politics' of truth: that is the type of discourse it accepts and makes function as true; the mechanisms and instances which enable one to distinguish true and false statements, the means by which each is sanctioned: the techniques and procedures accorded value in the acquisition of truth; the status of those who are charged with saying what counts as true.
>
> (1980: 131)

### The emerging 'discourse' of youth work management

Looking back over the last decade it is not hard to find evidence of an emerging discourse of management which has come to colonize the professional field of youth work. There have been a number of recent publications of books on leadership and management, for example Ford et al. (2005), Harrison et al. (2007) and Tyler et al. (2009). We have also seen the development of National Occupational Standards for Youth Work (LLUK, 2008) in which two out of five 'first level functions' identified as 'key purposes of youth work' are directly to do with managing the work. The primary role of the occupational standards in facilitating the management of organizations rather the practice of youth work is explicit in the document:

> Our aim is that the standards are versatile and support employers in a range of ways, including:
>
> • Performance management (e.g. appraisals)
> • Identifying training needs
> • Aid in structuring learning programmes (formal and informal)
> • Recruitment and selection (e.g. job descriptions)
> • Assessing achievement
> • Formal recognition of competence (e.g. continuing professional development)
> • Careers guidance and counselling.
>
> (LLUK, 2008: 5)

The Children's Workforce Development Council (CWDC), in its strategy for the development of the young people's workforce, identified capacity building of managers as a priority. It commissioned the Hay Group to report on the training needs of the children's workforce, which produced the following recommendations:

1    a Children's Workforce integrated approach to leadership talent management;
2    a Children's Workforce management and leadership programme;
3    a Children's Workforce performance management process;
4    a single communication channel to middle managers relating to leadership training and development opportunities.

(CWDC, 2008)

CWDC then commissioned a national programme of training, delivered by the FPM Training Consortium, with the aim of developing the skills and knowledge associated with leading and managing youth work and services for young people. The attention, and the funding, being given to the activities of leading and managing by national bodies charged with the development of services to young people is instructive. It tells us about their belief in leading and managing as the practices which can transform youth work, making it more efficient and effective, but these initiatives can also be understood as constructing a discourse through which the profession comes to see itself as dependent on the capacities of leaders and managers in order to achieve its aims. As the promotional leaflet 'New Programmes for Leaders and Managers of Services to Young People' stated:

It is a once in a generation opportunity for leaders and managers across the whole of the youth workforce to work side by side to enhance their capacities so they can deliver distinctive and connected services which meet the needs of young people now.

(FPM Training, undated)

Here youth work practitioners are being urged towards solidarity, working side by side, in the cause of enhancing their capacities as leaders and managers in the cause of delivering services which better meet the needs of young people. The statement seeks to be persuasive by touching on themes which are often part of the discourse of youth workers. Working side by side, not only with each other but also with young people; identifying and meeting the needs of young people; these are aspects of the work which are frequently evoked in youth work circles. But these ideas about the nature of practice are being elided with the practices of leading and managing, so the reader is led to understand that it is only through developing capacities for leading and managing that these outcomes become achievable.

In its own list of achievements for the young people's workforce in the period 2005–2011, the Children's Workforce Development Council points to 'Over 5,500 leaders and managers in the young people's workforce [who] have been trained to deliver integrated youth support', stating:

One of the key strands for improvement to drive forward the change agenda is strengthening leadership and management. The aim is to ensure that, by the end of March 2011, those leading and managing youth services are supported so that they can deliver integrated services for young people. In turn this will also help to raise the competence and capacity of leadership and management in the young people's workforce.

(CWDC, 2010)

The cumulative effect of these pronouncements and initiatives is to establish a discourse which uncontroversially accepts the idea that expertise in leadership and management is the primary factor in determining the quality of services provided by professionals in this and other related fields. In the above quote 'improvement' and 'change' are *discursively* linked to 'strengthening leadership and management'. The result is a belief that the 'competence and capacity' of the workforce will be raised, necessarily delivering improved services for young people. Importantly, one of the achievements of this discourse is to displace or silence alternative discourses which might, for example, draw attention to the importance of practices which respect young people's community and cultural identities as a basis for improving services to young people (Davies, 2005). (The notion of alternative discourses is explored more in the following chapter.)

Foucault (1980) argues that power is inherent in discourse, since it is through discourse that 'regimes of truth' are established and meanings attached to contemporary developments. Wetherell (2001: 25) makes the point that 'control over discourse is a vital source of power'. In his critique of educational practices in schools, Stephen Ball points to the important ways in which discourses embody the effects of power by defining the limits of expression and imagination.

> Discourses are about what can be said and thought, but also about who can speak, when, and with what authority.
>
> (Ball, 1990: 2)

In the above, Ball draws attention to the role of discourse not just in constituting truths about the world, 'what can be said', but also the identities of those who can legitimately speak. This link between discourse, power and identity has been explored by a number of writers (Rose, 1996; du Gay, 1996; Harrison et al., 2003; Chappell et al., 2003). What they draw our attention to is the role of discourse in constructing certain kinds of 'subjects', for example youth work managers, who are seen as legitimate and authoritative. In their analysis of education and training courses Chappell et al. (2003) argue that all educational programmes aimed at personal and professional growth 'contain implicit theorisations concerning the nature of the self'. Basing their analysis on Foucault's notion of 'technologies of the self', they argue that 'educational and training programmes are best seen as technologies for constructing particular kinds of people or subjects' (2003: 10). As can be seen from our review of recent examples of government funded initiatives to reinvigorate the youth work profession, the subject in view has been that of the 'leader and manager', not the youth work practitioner. It is in this 'managerial' role that authority is currently being invested.

In the latter half of this chapter, we have examined the ways in which a discourse of management expertise presents itself as an objective and technically neutral mechanism, dedicated only to greater efficiency and effectiveness. The technical rational basis on which management rests its claim to authority offers the possibility of professionals gaining control of the complex processes inherent in their work, but it also constrains the scope of that work within the straitjacket of technical rationalism and the discipline of auditing and accountability. It exerts powerful instrumental pressures towards uniformity, as management techniques become applied across contexts of practice.

The intention of deploying a postmodern critique in this chapter is not to deny or belittle the value of many of the 'capacity building' innovations introduced over recent years, but to step back from the persuasive and pervasive discourse of efficiency and effectiveness which they promote, and ask how far contemporary accounts of leading and managing actually support the professional identities and values, as well as the principles and practices, which underpin youth work.

## Conclusion

It is argued that a theoretical grounding is essential to enable an informed understanding of management principles and practices in youth work. Too often the dominant perspective is portrayed, not only as rational and taken for granted, but as the only approach. This managerialist approach often runs counter to the principles and practices of youth work (Smith, 2003; Ord, 2004; 2007; Davies and Merton, 2009). It is suggested that the theoretical grounding and the development of alternative ways of conceptualizing management processes, whether that be from a modernist or postmodernist perspective, would enable both practitioners and managers to not only resist the negative elements of managerialism but also to develop practices that both embrace youth work and allow it to develop and flourish.

## Questions for reflection and discussion

1   What are the relative merits of each of the mainstream management theories?
2   How might humanistic management practices improve youth work management?
3   How has a dominant 'discourse' of management affected both how managers are seen, and how managers operate, within youth work organizations, and how might this discourse be challenged?

## Further reading

### For 'mainstream' management theory

Mullins, L. J. (2007) *Management and Organisational Behaviour* (8th edn) Harlow: Financial Times/Prentice Hall.

### Readings for postmodern management

Alvesson, M. and Willmott, H. (1996) *Making Sense of Management: A Critical Introduction*, London: Sage.
Parker, M. (2000) 'Postmodernising organisation behaviour: new organisations or new organisational theory?' In J. Barry, J. Chandler, H. Clark, R. Johnston and D. Needle (eds) *Organisation and Management: A Critical Text*, London: Thomson Business Press, pp. 36–50.

## References

Banks, S. (2010) *Ethical Issues in Youth Work* (2nd edn) Abingdon: Routledge.
Ball, S. (1990) 'Introduction', in Ball, S. (ed.) *Foucault and Education: Disciplines and Knowledge*, London: Routledge, pp. 1–8.

Bracy, M. (2007) 'The accidental leader', in R. Harrison, C. Benjamin, S. Curran and R. Hunter (eds) *Leading Work with Young People*, London: Sage, pp. 25–33.

Chappell, C., Rhodes, C., Solomon, N., Tennant, M. and Yates, L. (2003) *Reconstructing the Lifelong Learner: Pedagogy and Identity in Individual, Organisational and Social Change*, London: Routledge.

Clarke, J. (1998) 'Doing the right thing? Managerialism and social welfare', in P. Abbot and L. Meerabeau (eds) *The Sociology of the Caring Professions* (2nd edn) London: UCL Press, pp. 234–51.

Clarke, J., Gewirtz, S. and McClaughlin, E. (eds) (2000) *New Managerialism, New Welfare*, London: Sage/Open University Press.

Cole, G. (2004) *Management Theory and Practice* (6th edn) London: Thomson Learning.

Cooper, R. and Burrell, G. (1988) 'Modernism, postmodernism and organisational analysis: an introduction', *Organisational Studies*, 9(1): 91–112.

CWDC (Children's Workforce Development Council) (2008) *Report: The Training and Development of Middle Managers in the Children's Workforce*, https://www.cwdcouncil.org.uk/assets/0000/8597/Web09_Training_and_development_for_middle_managers_report.pdf (accessed 20/2/11).

——(2010) 'Achievements of the last five years', http://www.cwdcouncil.org.uk/top-achievements (accessed 23/12/10).

Davies, B. (2005) 'Youth work: a manifesto for our times', *Youth and Policy*, no. 88, Summer: 5–27.

Davies, B. and Merton, B. (2009) 'Squaring the circle? The state of youth work in some children and young people's services', *Youth and Policy*, no. 103, Summer: 5–24.

DfCSF (2007) *Aiming High for Young People: A Ten Year Strategy for Positive Activities*, London: HMSO.

DfES (2002) *Transforming Youth Work: Resourcing Excellent Youth Services*, London: HMSO.

——(2003) *Every Child Matters*, London: HMSO.

Doyle, M. E. (1999) 'Called to be an informal educator', *Youth and Policy*, no. 65, Autumn: 28–37.

du Gay, P. (1996) *Consumption and Identity at Work*, London: Sage.

Edwards, P. K. and Scullion, H. (1982) *The Social Organisation of Industrial Conflict*, Oxford: Basil Blackwell.

Edwards, R. (2001) 'Meeting individual learner needs: power, subject, subjection', in C. Paechter, M. Preedy, D. Scott and J. Soler (eds) *Knowledge, Power and Learning*, London: Sage, pp. 37–46.

Farnham, D. and Horton, S. (eds) (1993) *Managing the New Public Services*, Basingstoke: Macmillan.

Ford, K., Hunter, R., Merton, B. and Waller, D. (2005) *Leading and Managing Youth Work and Youth Services for Young People*, Leicester: NYA.

Foucault, M. (1977) *Discipline and Punish: The Birth of the Prison*, London: Penguin.

——(1980) *Power/Knowledge: Selected Interviews and Other Writings 1972–1977*, Brighton: Harvester.

FPM Training (undated) 'New Programmes for Leaders and Managers of Services for Young People', Leicester: FPM.

Gordon, C. (1994) 'Introduction', in J. D. Faubion (ed.) *Power: Essential Works of Foucault 1954–1984, Volume 3*, London: Penguin, pp. xi–xli.

Handy, C. (1999) *Understanding Organisations* (4th edn) London: Pelican.

Hannagan, T. (2008) *Management: Concepts and Practices*, London: Prentice Hall.

Harrison, R., Benjamin, C., Curran, S. and Hunter, R. (eds) (2007) *Leading Work with Young People*, London: Sage.

Harrison, R., Clarke, J., Reeve, F. and Edwards, R. (2003) 'Doing identity work: fuzzy boundaries and flexibility in further education', *Research in Post-Compulsory Education*, 8(1): 105–17.

Kotter, J. P. (1996) *Leading Change*, New York: Harvard Business School Press.

Jeffs, T. and Smith, M. K. (2005) *Informal Education: Conversation, Democracy and Learning* (3rd edn) Nottingham: Education Heretics Press.

Likert, R. (1961) *New Patterns of Management*, London: McGraw-Hill.

LLUK (2008) *National Occupational Standards for Youth Work*, London: LLUK.

Maslow, A. (1954) *Motivation and Personality*, London: Harper and Row.

Mintzberg, H. (1973) *The Nature of Managerial Work*, London: Harper and Row.

Mullins, L. J. (2007) *Management and Organisational Behaviour*, (8th edn) Prentice Hall.

Nicholl, K. and Harrison, R. (2003) 'Constructing the good teacher in higher education: the discursive work of standards', *Studies in Continuing Education*, 25(1): 23–35.

Ord, J. (2004) 'The youth work curriculum as process not as output and outcome to aid accountability', *Youth and Policy*, no. 85: 53–69.

——(2007) *Youth Work Process, Product and Practice: Creating an Authentic Curriculum in Work with Young People*, Lyme Regis: RHP.

Parker Follett, M. (1940) *Dynamic Administration: The Collected Papers of Mary Parker Follett*, eds H. C. Metcalf and L. Urwick, New York: Harper.

Rose, N. (1996) *Inventing Ourselves: Psychology, Power, Personhood*, Cambridge: Cambridge University Press.

Schein, E. H. (1965) *Organizational Psychology*, Boston: Allyn and Bacon.

Smith, M. K. (1988) *Developing Youth Work*, Milton Keynes: Open University Press.

——(2003) 'From youth work to youth development', *Youth and Policy*, no. 79, Spring: 46–59.

Soreide, G. E. (2007) 'The public face of teacher identity: narrative construction of teacher identity in public policy documents', *Journal of Education Policy*, 22(2): 129–46.

Taylor, F. (1947) *Scientific Management*, London: Harper and Row.

Tyler, M., Hoggarth, L. and Merton, B. (2009) *Managing Modern Youth Work*, Exeter: Learning Matters.

Wetherell, M. (2001) 'Themes in discourse research: the case of Diane', in M. Wetherell, S. Taylor and S. J. Yates (eds) *Discourse Theory and Practice: A Reader*, London: Sage, pp. 14–28.

Young, K. (2005) *The Art of Youth Work* (2nd edn) Lyme Regis: RHP.

**Part II**

# Critical issues in the practice of youth work management

# 4 On managerial discourses, cultures and structures

## Pat Fuller and Jon Ord

Following on from the previous chapter which discussed the importance of postmodern ideas about 'discourse', this chapter considers two more alternative 'critical' perspectives, namely 'labour process theory' and 'critical management studies'. Before going on to ask important questions about what would be an appropriate culture and structure for youth work management. It continues to suggest that practitioners and managers alike reflect on the persuasive and pervasive discourse of efficiency and effectiveness which is being promoted, and ask how far contemporary accounts of leading and managing support the values and principles which underpin youth work.

This first section considers the sociological analyses of the workplace which followed on from and critiqued the positivist and uncritical nature of the early mainstream approaches in management theory and industrial sociology. It traces the development of a 'structuralist' approach, which highlighted the importance of understanding organizations in the economic and political context in which they operate. It then considers poststructuralist studies which consider both the way in which the social context shapes organizations, and the significance of 'agency', the ability of individuals to influence, to resist, change and reshape their work environments and to critique and challenge dominant discourses. Though rarely discussed in the field of youth work management, these ideas nevertheless have characteristics that resonate with key features of youth work, and provide frameworks through which to develop critical analysis of management theory and practice. They take account of the changing nature of modern workplaces and consider organizations, labour relations and management in the wider context of society, history and politics.

'Labour process theory' and 'critical management studies' look at organizations from perspectives that are both different from, and critical of mainstream theory. In that, they open up ways of thinking about management that are particularly relevant to youth work. Amongst these are questions that have not always been central to mainstream management theory: how a diversity of voices and experiences can be heard, how democratic decision making can be protected and developed. They are also critical of mainstream management theory that disregards social structure and the political and economic context, as well as its scant basis in empirical evidence, and the way in which cultures and identities at work are formed, and developed, over time.

## Labour process theory

Labour process theory focuses on the contested nature of the relationship between managers and the workforce. It made what Burawoy (2008) describes as a radical break with the earlier work in industrial sociology that informed mainstream management theory, and did so from a Marxist 'structuralist' perspective. It explicitly challenged the way in which industrial relations had been understood by suggesting that the organization of work, in capitalist production, led to the management of the workplace in ways which led to increasing control and subordination of the workforce (Braverman, 1974). It opened the way to extensive research studies into management and labour relations (Friedman, 1977; Pollert, 1981; Edwards and Scullion, 1982; Brown, 1992) which were characterized by detailed studies of the workplace and increasingly complex analyses of the nature of management and of work. A good example of this is Burawoy (1979) who, working as a machine operator in an Allied Corporation factory, undertook detailed ethnographic, participant observation studies of the ways in which workers responded to managers' assertion of what Clarke (1998) later referred to as the 'right to manage'. His study revealed the complexity of 'resistance' and 'conflict' which underlies worker–manager relations. It identified the subtle 'compensatory logic' of establishing routines which enabled employees to control some of their own workloads, and the 'game playing' which enabled them to mediate power relationships in the workplace.

He describes his interest as stemming from an article by Antonio Gramsci, 'Americanism and Fordism', in which the Italian Marxist observes of the USA, 'hegemony here is born in the factory' (Burawoy, 1979: xii). His work highlighted the significance of the political structures within which organizations operate, as well as how power relationships are shaped. He suggested that the 'importance of the everyday life of the shopfloor' is a critical element in understanding how 'manufacturing consent' in the workplace occurs (Burawoy, 1979: 191).

Ackroyd and Thompson explore how and why conventional management theory rarely acknowledges conflict and resistance in workplace relationships, except in relation to the management of change or in specialist work on conflict resolution. They note how perceptions of 'management' are socially constructed, and draw attention to the lack of empirical evidence of what managers actually do and of how everyday practice is experienced in workplaces. 'Paradoxical though it may seem, what organizational behaviour is like in its ordinary forms has not been subjected to considerable analysis and discussion' (Ackroyd and Thompson, 1999: 9). The possibility has also not been considered, that resistance and conflict is a rational response to inappropriate managerial practices. This is notably true of youth work, where everyday conflict and issues over power and decision making appear to be no less common than they are in workplaces in general. Ironically, since the advent of 'managerialism', which has exacerbated conflict between managers and practitioners, little attention has been given to everyday aspects of the reality of management and there has been little detailed observation and research.

Importantly, the structuralist and poststructuralist perspectives in labour process theory and the resulting critical management studies, see the dynamic of the worker–manager relationship in a completely different way, fundamentally challenging the dominant discourse and the perceived 'right to manage'. They attempt to undermine existing top-down power relations and work towards supplanting them with more democratic relationships and structures. In addition, this perspective questions the dominant assumptions within managerialism *that resistance can and ought to be 'managed out'*. Not only is this quite probably not possible, but ultimately, many (including the 'humanist' theorists we saw in Chapter 3), argue that the 'effectiveness' of any organization must be grounded in the degree to which workers and managers 'work together' to commonly agreed goals (O'Doherty and Willmott, 2001). Furthermore it could equally be argued that 'dissent is an essential component of intellectual and social progress' (Gilchrist et al., 2011: vi) and at the heart of successful democratic processes.

A further critique of mainstream management theory has focused on the extent to which the wider social and political context within which management theory is developed and practised has been sacrificed in the desire to find universal generalized models of effectiveness. Burawoy's (2008) observation that 1974, the year of publication of Braverman's *Labor and Monopoly Capital*, was also a time of major recession, the rise of neoliberalism, a shift from production to service industries and the year in which 'union density in the public sector first exceeded union density in the private sector' (2008: 372) in the USA. This confirms how important it can be to understand the historical and economic background to particular theories, practices and discourses. In more recent times the organization of work in many fields has been changing, rapidly, and sometimes dramatically. As we saw in Chapter 2, the influence of the neoliberal 'modernizing' agenda emphasizing both privatization and the three E's (of efficiency, effectiveness and economy, Farnham and Horton, 1996) has had a profound influence on organizations in the public and voluntary sectors in the UK. Most recently, the implication of this has been the rise of commissioning, and youth work being delivered through social enterprise and community interest companies under contract.

## Critical management theory

A separate but equally important 'critical' approach to the conceptualization of management is encompassed within the growing body of 'critical management theory' (Deetz, 1992; Morgan, 1990; Alvesson and Willmott, 2003; Clegg et al., 2005). This sets out to 'combine the respective strengths of philosophical and empirical modes of investigation' (Alvesson and Willmott, 1992: 17). It attempts to develop an approach, which draws from Habermas and Foucault, to question the assumed 'neutrality of management and the impartiality of management practice' and to explore power relationships within organizations (Alvesson and Willmott, 1992: 4), key themes of which are the critique of the discourse of mainstream management theory (as introduced in Chapter 3), and of the scarcity of evidence on which much of that theory is based.

Clegg et al. (2005) describe how the use of power by managers is seen as an everyday reality, exclusively concerned with how management can exercise power more effectively or more comprehensively. This may not only be ethically questionable but also have implications that make it ineffective, particularly in facilitating the influence of a multiplicity of voices and democratic decision making. In youth work, setting managerial targets, for example, requires workers to be accountable to a predefined set of criteria for their work, but also creates a form of surveillance in which staff become, in effect, responsible for 'policing' their own work, and reduces opportunities for them to 'think differently', work autonomously and contribute to strategic planning.

The central themes of critical management studies are:

- questioning assumptions about management,
- highlighting the influence of power and ideology,

- challenging technicist claims to rationality, and
- working for more democratic and just organizations.

Rigg and Trehan (1999)

Critical management studies has opened up spaces for feminist, anti-oppressive and environmentalist critiques of mainstream management theory and for work on possibilities for more inclusive and diverse management practice.

Martin (2003) suggests that the question of how feminist understandings of the interrelationship between gender, 'race' and class inequalities can bring breadth to studies of women in management. Previously such studies have largely focused on the existence of 'glass ceilings', preventing the promotion of women to higher management roles, rather than wider and more significant questions such as 'whose voices' are excluded from decision making. This has led to more radical investigation of ways in which exclusion operates within management through the representation of the interests of men, and of managers, and can be represented in mainstream theory as universal, hence 'silencing the voices and ignoring the interests of women' (Martin, 2003: 68). Furthermore, the feminist deconstruction of concepts and dichotomies that Martin cites, particularly those of 'male and female, objectivity and subjectivity, competition and cooperation, and rationality and emotionality' (2003: 67), can raise questions about the 'taken for granted' realities of organizational structures and cultures.

Rigg and Trehan's (1999) study of management education suggests that the concept of the learning 'community' can be problematic, and has often been presented naively. Even core values of organizational development, such as openness and honesty, are called into question by the imbalances of power, status and social/cultural capital that exist within groups that are mixed in race, gender and class terms. Under the title 'Not Critical Enough?', their work raises the question of whether critical management studies has itself been seduced by the desire to find one size that fits all. For youth work, which, it can be argued, has been shaped by the influences of divergent voices, and for which equality of opportunity has been a strong and persistent theme, the question of how management can be democratic and inclusive is of fundamental importance.

The 'green' or environmental perspective is also articulated from within critical management studies and this offers a further challenge to how management respond to a separate but nonetheless equally important range of local and global priorities. Jermier and Forbes (2003) offer a critique of the range of management 'greening' initiatives in the private sector, which they characterize as regulatory, ceremonial, competitive or holistic. They argue that the traditional management view of organizations, with an emphasis on a unified organizational culture, fails to recognize and work with the contradictory elements of organizations. Drawing on the work of Herbert Marcuse in *One-Dimensional Man* (1964), they suggest that 'the integrative power of his critical analysis can help students of management think more systematically about the macro forces in contemporary society' (Jermier and Forbes, 2003: 158). They also cite Sinclair (1993), arguing:

> The strength of any organization is found in its subcultural pluralism, especially when it comes to ethical decision-making. This is because being ethical requires ongoing self-examination and deep reflection and these processes are enhanced

from the discourse about values that is inevitable when subcultural diversity is respected.

(Jermier and Forbes, 2003: 170–71)

## On structures:

Mullins defines an organization's structure as: 'the pattern of relationships among positions in the organization and among members of the organization' (2007: 564). There is no doubt that structures are important. Structure gives a form to the organization and according to Mullins it 'makes possible the application of the process of management and creates a framework of order ... through which the activities of the organization can be planned, organized, directed and controlled' (ibid.). Whilst much of this might be the case, there is little doubt that structures are, in the main, conceptualized in a top-down hierarchical manner, in order to cascade the authority of the principal officer or chief executive through the organization – as evidenced by the emphasis on 'control and order'.

Mullins points out that 'it is essential to give full attention to the structure and design of an organization' (2007: 590). Whilst clearly acknowledging that this is not always an easy task, and accepting that there are technical requirements, Mullins however goes on to argue that 'consideration should be given to social factors, and that the needs and demands of the human part of the organization [are necessary] to encourage the willing participation of members' (ibid.). However, it is important to draw a distinction between organizational form and organizational behaviour, that is, between what the organization 'looks like' and how the organization is represented, and what the organization and, more importantly, the people within it, 'actually do'.

Too often this distinction is ignored and managers make the mistake of assuming that a necessary link exists between structure and action, a mistaken belief that if only they get the structure right everything else will fall into place. As Heller reminds us: 'No amount of reorganizing and reshuffling will increase the long-term capability of a business unless you suit the organization to the people and to a genuinely shared purpose' (1996: 21). It is argued that a manager who places too much emphasis on structures is being too 'scientific', seeing the organization as a rational project, and attempting to create the 'best' pattern and arrangement of the organization independent of the people within it. Again Heller points out:

> Neat structural organization and good management are not synonymous ... [we] saw that true organization wasn't about structure, but about increasing long-term capability ... That hinges fundamentally on people and relationships between them.

(1996: 21)

Whilst structures can create easily identifiable patterns of line management responsibility, delineate working groups, and give shape and form to the organization, both internally and to external stakeholders, structures can as easily create division and separation, and decrease, rather than increase, the communication across the organization, more often than not stifling creativity and innovation rather than facilitating it.

Arguably the dominant structure within youth work organizations, certainly large local authority youth services and the larger voluntary organizations, is a hierarchical structure. The universal acceptance of 'the right to manage' has done little to question the adoption of this dominant pattern of organizational structure. This is most commonly reflected in the following hierarchical pattern (Figure 4.1):

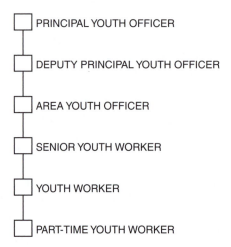

*Figure 4.1* A typical youth service structure (Bradford and Day, 1991: 32)

Hierarchical and bureaucratic structures place an over-emphasis on line management relationships. Bradford and Day suggest that this: 'oversimplifies organizational life and ignores the potential for a variety of managerial roles and relationships, and ... intensifies accountability' (1991: 33). They go on to suggest that functions such as monitoring and supervising workers need not be the exclusive role of line managers (see Chapter 8 for an exploration of this). Similarly the role of coordinating and leading particular projects is hindered, rather than developed, by the rigid divisions that line management and hierarchical bureaucracies produce. Bradford and Day's research also suggested that formal line management structures do not actually facilitate decision making, as, for example, whilst in theory an area youth worker was: 'supposed to be responsible to the deputy principal. It all gets confused because the principal comes straight to us with things ... and if I'm honest we tend to go straight to him if there's a problem. The Deputy gets stuck in the middle' (1991: 29). Similarly Bradford and Day found that there was also a problem with youth workers: 'getting decisions about things – money, equipment, and so on' (ibid.), often resulting in youth workers needing to go further up the chain for a decision, leading them to question levels of the bureaucracy: 'I don't know why we have team leaders' (ibid.).

Such criticisms lead to a questioning of the overriding dominance of hierarchical and bureaucratic structures. Interestingly, Lord Sugar, CEO and chairman of the very successful company Amstrad, has quite a different perspective on structures:

> There are no formal management structures in my companies; much to the disapproval of many. I know what is going on partly because I have told people what to do, and ensured the team is in place to deliver, and partly because I ask what is going on. It is not always easy to implement, but in theory it really is that simple.
>
> (2005: 90)

*Alternative structures*

Interestingly, Mullins notes, the business sector is beginning to question the traditional structures of organizations as: 'companies face increasing global competitiveness and complex demands ... the need arises for alternative forms of corporate structure' (2007: 50). He suggests this has led to a questioning of the traditional hierarchy, and a move towards 'more decentralised flatter structures' (ibid.). He defines a flat structure as having: 'broad spans of control and few levels of authority' (Mullins 2007: 804). Mullins goes on to suggest that: 'If an organization values individual development, open communication and trust, it lends itself to flat, open and networked structures' (Mullins 2007: 178). It is argued that in youth work which places a great deal of emphasis on the autonomy of the practitioner to respond to the needs of young people in innovative and creative ways, the structures within which the work is located must be ones that best facilitate cooperation, communication and responsiveness. It is evident that youth work managers need to think more creatively about how their organizations are structured.

Mullins does note that in a flat structure, as a span of control is widened the chain of command is correspondingly weakened. Clearly flatter structures present a challenge to the managerialism which places a great emphasis on control and command styles of management. Similarly flatter structures require an element of trust in employees as the controls begin to diminish, a point that will be returned to shortly as we reflect upon the importance of culture. It is also worth pausing for a moment and considering the possibility of establishing more radical alternatives, such as a cooperative structure. While certainly not common in youth work organizations, neither is it entirely absent. There are some interesting if isolated examples of innovative structures which are entirely democratic. These share positions of authority, for example with a rotating chair at meetings, and each member of the organization has equal status and rights. Interestingly a specific example of this type of managerial practice, perhaps not surprisingly, occurred in a women's refuge. This profoundly echoes some of the earlier critiques from critical management studies which argued for alternative ways of both valuing people in organizations and about how the practice of management should be enacted.

# On culture

Whilst arguably managers place too much emphasis on overt structures, the formal representation of the relationships between members of an organization, they probably place too little emphasis on cultural considerations. The culture of an organization is certainly as, if not more, important than its structure. We saw in the previous chapter how important the less tangible, but nonetheless profound impact of humanistic aspects of the management process have on workers' capabilities and performance: 'Elton Mayo's research revealed that every organization has an informal structure which affects how people behave, how the system functions and which management methods need to be adopted to raise morale and assist people to be mentally healthy at work' (Coulshed et al., 2006: 37). Elton Mayo's research into motivation demonstrated how productivity increased when workers felt attended to and respected, and this undermined the scientific and 'rational' approach to management. It is this humanistic, 'informal' aspect of the organization that in part underpins its culture.

Hannagan refers to an organization's culture as simply: 'the way we do things around here' (2008: 23). As such, culture relates to the often implicit and intangible aspects of an organization which are, however, no less important. Underpinned by the norms, values, assumptions and accepted practices within the organization, the culture has a profound influence on an organization and its management practices.

> Managerial work in any youth service is both influenced by and is an expression of its culture. Managers are involved in the design and implementation of an organization's systems, and it is important that they are clear about the values expressed through these systems. They should also be aware that their own managerial style and approach is an expression of values, whether personal or organizational, and will be interpreted as such by staff.
>
> (Bradford and Day, 1991: 22)

However, Ford et al. emphasise that 'rather than accepting the culture as a given, the effective manager will take steps to build and develop the culture that best fits the organization's purpose and values' (2005: 47). It is evident therefore that the culture of youth work organizations and the values which underpin them are of the utmost importance in how effective the organization will be.

An important feature of an organization's culture is established by the extent to which policy and procedure are formalized. Payne (1987: 66) distinguishes between organizations which produce 'detailed and lengthy policy documents' and those at the other extreme, where: 'policy is merely the accumulation of decisions made over the years, what might be called custom and practice' (ibid.). Arguably with the rise of managerialism there has been a distinct shift away from a culture based on 'custom and practice' to one which is dominated by increasingly detailed policy and procedures. Such policies and procedures Payne rightly argues can become: 'so rigid that little room is left [for] professional discretion ... and [such] inflexible controls may hamper development and innovation' (1987: 66).

If we accept, for a moment, Payne's basic definition of a manager as: 'anyone who has responsibility for the work of others' (1987: 71), he argues therefore that how a manager interprets this responsibility and how this in turn informs their managerial practices 'is a defining feature of organizational culture'. At the heart of how this responsibility is interpreted and applied are the notions of discretion and autonomy, as well as the type of accountability that emerges from how they are enacted in the organization. Payne uses McGregor's classic 'theory X' and 'theory Y' to illustrate two very different approaches to autonomy. 'Theory X' and 'theory Y' depict two opposing styles of management based upon differing beliefs about human nature and behaviour at work (Mullins, 2007: 444–46).

Theory X is based on a belief that people are extrinsically motivated to work, and require the carrot and stick approach: 'The central principle of theory X is direction and control through a centralized system of organization and the exercise of authority' (Mullins, 2007: 444). According to theory X workers are essentially demotivated to work, and need prescription, direction and strong managerial controls in order that organizational objectives can be fulfilled. Theory Y developed out of the humanistic school of management, has a more progressive view of work and the attitude of workers to it. It sees workers as far more intrinsically motivated and believes: 'people will exercise self direction and self-control in the service of objectives to which they are committed' (ibid.). According to theory Y work is an integral part of life and fulfils a number of needs beyond basic security. Workers therefore have a commitment to their work and to the organization.

Importantly, Mullins favours theory Y, suggesting that it: 'represents the assumptions consistent with current research knowledge' (2007: 444). Whilst perhaps no manager or organizational culture is entirely depicted by theory Y or theory X, arguably, cultures do gravitate towards one or the other. The bottom line is whether the manager trusts the workers or not. The extent to which managers gravitate towards theory X or theory Y in practice will depend on the balance between the 'discretion' given to the workers and the 'limits' prescribed by the manager. Discretion refers to 'the necessary choices and judgements that individuals must make when working ... The prescribed limits are the boundaries which are set around work: policies, rules, procedures, methods, and so on ... confirming what is required of the individual worker' (Bradford and Day, 1991: 13). Evidently with the rise of managerialism, 'prescribed limits' have increased and youth workers are experiencing unparalleled controls, whilst at the same time the degree of discretion afforded to youth workers is increasingly limited.

Interestingly, research conducted in the 1980s by Bradford and Day found a very different situation: 'in the youth service, these elements are often unclear'. They suggest workers were often very unclear about what expectations managers had of them: 'no one's ever said anything about how the work here should be done', or 'I think the work of the Centre is okay because nobody, the management committee or the youth officer, hasn't said anything ... but they haven't said what sort of thing they expect anyway ... ' (1991: 14). Similarly: 'I have been here 18 months now and nobody has ever checked on me to see how I am doing. I think I'm doing what is expected but I couldn't be sure' (1991: 27). Similarly Smith, commenting on local authority reviews of youth work, notes that: 'services and workers were confused about their aims and objectives. Policies and priorities were non-existent, unclear, confused or made irrelevant by the passage of time and changing circumstances' (Smith, D. I., 1987, cited in Jeffs and Smith, 1988: 235).

It is hard to believe a youth worker in the twenty-first century could experience such 'hands off' management. However, even up until the 1980s the type of management youth workers experienced certainly appeared to have more in common with the notion of manager as 'advisor' as outlined by Davies in Chapter 1, where minimal controls were exercised, and a high degree of trust and discretion was afforded to individual workers. Characteristic also of the culture of youth work at that time, however, was also a: 'deep-seated resistance to management ... both to being managers and to being managed' (Millar, 1995: 49). Whilst Jeffs and Smith suggest that this 'frontier spirit ... may lead to a rich diversity of practice' (1988: 236), questions of accountability were entirely absent.

Many of the following chapters of this book chart a number of the ways in which managerialism has impacted on youth work practice, including planning, evaluation and supervision, as well as across both centre-based and detached youth work. Managerialism has placed an overriding importance on exercising accountability and ensuring youth work responds to policy directives. As a result the pendulum of managerial control has significantly swung away from autonomy and discretion towards command and control. Undoubtedly theory X has infiltrated and infected the managerial practices of youth work.

## Towards a democratic culture in youth work management

The current climate of managerialism in youth work management is perhaps best illustrated as a clash of cultures. Youth work has a distinctive 'occupational culture'. Millar argues: 'key features of that culture included a concern with person centred approaches, a belief to promote active involvement in decision-making and the notion of the worker as an activist and campaigner' (2010: 133). Youth work organizations traditionally reflect youth work values of respect and self-determination (NYA, 2001) and dialogue, democracy and fostering learning (Jeffs and Smith, 2005). The cultural shift associated with managerialism runs counter to youth work values and firmly places workers as subordinate to managers through rigid line management and formalized hierarchies. This is evidenced further by the imposition of top-down targets, and formalized plans which identify priorities for workers independent of genuine needs analysis.

As was previously argued, senior managers have a critical role to play in making sure the organization is clear about its values and in managing in ways that reinforce those values (Ford et al., 2005: 90). However, the extent to which managers acquiesce to the dominant neoliberal culture, and impose this upon youth work, rather than challenge it and try to develop a culture which accords with youth work values, must be questioned.

### *Voice*

One of the ways in which the managerial culture could be improved would be to ensure the voice of youth workers is heard. Whilst it is accepted that: 'Where an organization encourages positive approaches to listening and responding to young people, youth work is likely to flourish' (Millar, 2010: 136), the issue of how well an organization is built around a diversity of voices is of particular importance. Craig et al. (2008), in their mapping of voluntary sector work with children and young people, note that

> Listening to the views of children and young people was seen as very important to all the organizations interviewed: 'it's at the core of what we do': but experience was patchy.
>
> (Craig et al., 2008: 65)

Davies (2010) could still find some evidence of the value of young people's voice and influence in current provision, but youth workers expressed concern that organizations were becoming more hierarchical and managers were struggling to keep up their contact with and support for their staff. His research suggests that policy directives and uncertainty about the future basis of the work had created a precarious situation in which both managers and staff alike felt that organizations were changing: becoming less responsive and less democratic, more concerned with their own internal mechanisms and, this would suggest, less able to be the kind of inclusive organization in which all, including young people's, voices, could genuinely be heard.

Harper notes that: 'part-time workers are largely excluded from discussion and decision-making processes, which results in an inevitable sense of alienation' (Harper, 1985: 15, cited in Jeffs and Smith, 1988: 234), and in organizations where a considerable amount of face-to-face work with young people is undertaken by part-time youth workers, they must be more involved. Questions must also be asked about how the involvement of young people is more than mere tokenism, or perhaps at best framed as 'active' participation in a consumerist model of feedback from service users. Members of the wider community also need to be acknowledged within the overall network of organizational communication. With the decline of management committees as legitimate forums for both the discussion, and identification, of priorities for youth work (Ord, 2011) a vital conduit to the community needs to be re-established (the community context of youth work is explored further in Chapter 9).

The context of integrated services within which youth work is increasingly operating is likely to further exacerbate the centralization of decision making and increase the focus on managerial control. In their research on youth work in integrated settings, Davies and Merton (see Chapter 11) convey a situation in which, though managers appeared to be more positive than workers about the future, they are still faced with stark choices. For some, comments like 'I'm not so much pressurised as powerless' and 'We're managing more by stealth … We know what we want to deliver (as youth workers) and how but we're less and less upfront about it' (Davies, 2010: 53, 55).

Despite the numerous policy constraints with which youth work management need to grapple, as has been previously argued within 'labour process' theory, resistance should not be seen as irrational and needing to be managed out. It is a rational response to the dominant discourse of inequality. Such dissent therefore needs to be incorporated into democratic managerial processes, as it contains legitimate concerns and points of view. Similarly critical management studies reflects the importance of the need to incorporate the disparate voices of the organization and wider society as well as the need to address the oppressive tendencies of dominant discourses.

### Relationships

Improvements in the culture of youth work management could also be made with acknowledgement of the importance of relationships. These are not only fundamental to youth work practice (Young, 2005; Ord, 2007). As Twelvetrees reminds us, they are equally important between the manager and youth worker, emphasizing: 'the importance of building relationships at all levels, upwards, downwards and laterally' (1987: 52). Good relationships between all levels of organization would ensure that managers understood the concerns and priorities of youth workers, as well as help to ensure the worker understands the constraints within which the manager is operating, as: 'such people are often under pressure themselves, from council committees and politicians for example and know that if a mistake is made, the youth service budget may suffer' (ibid.).

Too often the dominant managerial discourse creates a culture where: 'staff are treated as if they are incapable of thinking for themselves … ' (Mullins, 2007: 693). A return to a culture where respect is afforded to everyone in the organization regardless of their role, relationships are fostered, and voices are heard, would go some way to establish a viable culture of youth work management.

### Trust

Perhaps at the heart of a viable culture, however, is the issue of trust. The neoliberal agenda has consistently undermined professionals and 'professionalism'. Gone are the:

historic forms of professional management in which the professional was trained to a high level and largely to use his or her judgement in the delivery of services. This can be characterised as a shift from trust me (I am a professional) to prove it (and if you cannot I will sue).

(Ford et al., 2005: 110)

There is arguably a growing armoury of mechanisms which are intended to regulate professional activity, making it more accountable to central government and user groups, indicative of the changing perceptions of the place of professionals in society (Eraut, 1994). Central to this is the move from a model of high trust and low levels of external regulation of professional activity towards one of low trust and high levels of external regulation.

It should be remembered that trust is of fundamental importance. As O'Neill (2002) reminds us:

It isn't only rulers and governments who prize and need trust. Each of us and every profession and every institution needs trust ... The culture of accountability that we are relentlessly building for ourselves actually damages trust rather than supporting it. Plants don't flourish when we pull them up too often to check how their roots are growing: political institutional and professional life too may not go well if we constantly uproot them to demonstrate that everything is transparent and trustworthy.

Importantly, managerialism has been a structural as well as an ideological change, and some recent studies in other areas have begun detailed observational research on the impact of these changes on the organization of work. Angela McRobbie's (2002) preliminary study of radical changes in the cultural industries, notes the difficulty of sustaining workplace democracy and participation in decision making. She suggests that the new organizational contracts may serve to reinforce existing inequalities, injustice, oppression and discriminatory practice or, at the least, to make them more covert and harder to address. For the growing number of social enterprises in youth work, on commissioned contracts as well as those in the setting of integrated services, it is likely that most will reflect traditional management discourses and power relations and not be dedicated to finding ways of creating organizational decision making structures which genuinely reflect a diversity of perspectives amongst staff, the young people, and the communities that they serve. And those commissioning youth work find it more difficult in practice than in theory, to ensure that participative decision making and rights at work are protected.

It should be remembered that youth workers are in the vast majority of cases highly motivated and committed individuals who prioritize the needs of young people. A culture of management must be established which is based upon 'respect' for them as professionals, and needs to enable the 'disparate' voice of practitioners, and young people to be heard. The culture also needs to embed 'trust'. Clearly this is not a blind 'faith' and we are not advocating a return to the laissez-faire approach which Bradford and Day (1991) identified in the 1980s, but 'discretion and autonomy' need to be returned to their rightful place in the process of management.

*To conclude*, we cannot simply import management models from other industries, (as we have seen, even the corporate sector is questioning traditional management structures and cultures) not least because if youth work management is to be consistent with its values it needs to develop a culture which reflects those values rather than one which runs counter to them. 'Youth work operates at the informal, less structured end of the spectrum of work with young people, and it needs managers who recognise and build on its strengths rather than constrain it within an occupational straitjacket' (Millar, 2010: 144). Labour process theory reminds us of the importance of resistance, addressing issues of power and disempowerment. Critical management theory also raises important questions about hearing the many and varied voices of both practitioners, young people and the wider community. In order to manage youth work, managers need to be aware of, and work with the existing occupational culture of youth work. They must adopt management strategies to fit their circumstances, develop a culture which is respectful and trusts its workforce, and, more importantly, is democratic.

## Questions for reflection and discussion

1   Can you begin to identify which voices are silenced (or not heard) within the management process of youth work organizations?
2   How can we begin to ensure that disparate voices, and concerns, of the disempowered are engaged with in the management of youth work organizations?
3   What structures best enable the youth work values of democracy to be enacted?
4   Can you begin to identify what the aspects of a viable youth work culture are?

## Further reading

Alvesson, M. and Wilmott, H. (2003) *Studying Management Critically*, London: Sage.
Burawoy, M. (2008) 'The public turn: from labor process to labor movement', *Work and Occupations*, 35(4): 371–87.
Millar, G. (2010) 'Managing and developing youth work', in Jeffs, T. and Smith, M. K. (eds) *Youth Work Practice*, Basingstoke: Palgrave Macmillan.
O'Neill, O. (2002) 'Without trust we cannot stand', Reith lecture no. 1, www.bbc.co.uk/radio4/reith2002/lecture1.shtml (accessed 3 March 2011).
For a good example of the creation of a discourse, and how this limits how youth work is both conceived and delivered, see Hoyle, D. (2008) 'Problematizing Every Child Matters', *The Encyclopaedia of Informal Education*, available at www.infed.org/socialwork/every_child_matters_a_critique.htm

## References

Ackroyd, S. and Thompson, P. (1999) *Organizational Misbehaviour*, London: Sage.
Alvesson, M. and Willmott, H. (1992) *Critical Management Studies*, London: Sage.
——(2003) *Studying Management Critically*, London: Sage.
Bradford, S. and Day, M. (1991) *Youth Service Management: Aspects of Structure, Organisation, and Development*, Leicester: Youth Work Press/National Youth Agency.
Braverman, H. (1974) *Labor and Monopoly Capital*, New York: Monthly Review Press.
Brown, R. (1992) *Understanding Industrial Organisations: Theoretical Perspectives in Industrial Sociology*, London: Routledge.
Burawoy, M. (1979) *Manufacturing Consent*, Chicago: University of Chicago Press.
——(2008) 'The public turn: from labor process to labor movement', *Work and Occupations*, 35(4): 371–87.

Clark, J. (1998) 'Doing the right thing? Managerialism and social welfare', in Abbot, P. and Meerabeau, L. (eds) *The Sociology of the Caring Professions* (2nd edn) London: UCL Press, 234–51.

Clarke, J., Gewirtz, S. and McClaughlin, E. (eds) (2000) *New Managerialism, New Welfare*, London: Sage/Open University Press.

Clegg, S., Kornberger, M. and Pitsis, T. (2005) *Managing and Organizations: An Introduction to Theory and Practice*, London: Sage.

Cole, G. (2004) *Management Theory and Practice* (6th edn) London: Thomson Learning.

Coulshed, V. and Mullender, A., with Jones, D. N. and Thomson, N. (2006) *Management in Social Work*, Basingstoke: Palgrave Macmillan.

Craig, G., Gibson, H., Perkins, N., Wilkinson, M. and Wray, J. (2008) *Every Organisation Matters*, London: NCVCCO and NCVYS.

Davies, B. (2010) 'Straws in the wind: The state of youth work practice in a changing policy environment', *Youth and Policy*, Winter, no. 105: 9–36.

Davies, B. and Merton, B. (2009) 'Squaring the circle?: The state of youth work in some children and young people's services', *Youth and Policy*, Summer, no. 103: 5–24.

Deetz, S. (1992) *Democracy in an Age of Corporate Colonization: Developments in Communication and the Politics of Everyday Life*, Albany: State University of New York Press.

DfES (2003) *Every Child Matters*, London: HMSO.

Edwards, P. K. and Scullion, H. (1982) *The Social Organisation of Industrial Conflict*, Oxford: Basil Blackwell.

Eraut, M. (1994) *Developing Professional Knowledge and Competence*, London: Falmer Press.

Farnham, D. and Horton, S. (eds) (1996) *Managing the New Public Services* (2nd edn) London: Macmillan.

Ford, K., Hunter, R., Merton, B. and Waller, D. (2005) *Leading and Managing Youth Work and Youth Services for Young People*, Leicester: NYA.

Friedman, A. (1977) *Industry and Labour*, London: Macmillan.

Gilchrist, R., Hodgson, T., Jeffs, T., Spence, J., Stanton, N. and Walker, J. (2011) *Reflecting on the Past: Essays in History of Youth in Committee Work*, Lyme Regis: RHP.

Handy, C. (1999) *Understanding Organisations* (4th edn) London: Pelican.

Hannagan, T. (2008) *Management Concepts and Practices* (5th edn) London: Prentice Hall.

Heller, R. (1996) 'Resist that urge to reorganise', *Management Today*, January, p. 21.

Hoyle, D. (2008) 'Problematizing Every Child Matters', *The Encyclopaedia of Informal Education*, available at www.infed.org/socialwork/every_child_matters_a_critique.htm

Jeffs, T. and Smith, M. K. (1988) 'The promise of management of youth work', in Jeffs, T. and Smith, M. K. (eds) *Welfare and Youth Work Practice*, Basingstoke: Palgrave Macmillan, pp. 230–51.

——(2005) *Informal Education: Conversation, Democracy and Learning*, Nottingham: Education Heretics Press.

Jermier, J. M. and Forbes, L. (2003) 'Greening organisations: critical issues', in Alvesson, M. and Willmott, H. (eds) *Studying Management Critically*, London: Sage, pp. 157–175.

Kotter, J. P. (1996) *Leading Change*, New York: Harvard Business School Press.

Likert, R. (1961) *New Patterns of Management*, London: McGraw-Hill.

McRobbie, A. (2002) 'Clubs to companies: notes on the decline of political culture in speeded up creative worlds', *Cultural Studies*, 16(4): 516–31.

Marken, M. and Payne, M. (1988) *Enabling and Ensuring: Supervision in Practice*, Leicester: NYB.

Martin, J. (2003) 'Feminist theory and critical theory: unexplored synergies', in Alvesson, M. and Willmott, H. (eds) *Studying Management Critically*, London: Sage, pp. 66–91.

Maslow, A. (1954) *Motivation and Personality*, London: Harper and Row.

Millar, G. (1995) 'Beyond managerialism: an exploration of the occupational culture of youth and community work', *Youth and Policy*, Autumn, no. 50: 49–58.

——(2010) 'Managing and developing youth work', in Jeffs, T. and Smith, M. K. (eds) *Youth Work Practice*, Basingstoke: Palgrave Macmillan, pp. 133–44.

Mintzberg, H. (1973) *The Nature of Managerial Work*, London: Harper and Row.

Morgan, G. (1990) *Organizations in Society*, London: Macmillan.

Mullins, L. J. (2007) *Management and Organisational Behaviour* (8th edn) New Jersey: Prentice Hall.

NYA (2001) *Ethical Conduct in Youth Work: A Statement of Values and Principles*, Leicester: NYA.

O'Doherty, D. and Willmott, H. (2001) 'Debating labour process theory: the issue of subjectivity and the relevance of poststructuralism', *Sociology*, 35(2): 457–76.

O'Neill, O. (2002) 'Without trust we cannot stand', Reith lecture no. 1, www.bbc.co.uk/radio4/reith2002/lecture1.shtml (accessed 3 March 2011).

Ord, J. (2004) 'The youth work curriculum as process not as output and outcome to aid accountability', *Youth and Policy*, Autumn, no. 85: 53–69.

——(2007) *Youth Work Process, Product and Practice: Creating an Authentic Curriculum in Work with Young People*, Lyme Regis: RHP.

——(2011) 'The Kingston Youth Service: space, place and the Albermarle legacy', in Gilchrist, R., Hodgson, T., Jeffs, T., Spence, J., Stanton, N. and Walker, J. (eds) *Reflecting on the Past: Essays in History of Youth in Committee Work*, Lyme Regis: RHP, pp. 132–45.

Parker Follett, M. (1940) *Dynamic Administration: The Collected Papers of Mary Parker Follett*, eds Metcalf, H. C. and Urwick, L., New York: Harper.

Payne, M. (1987) 'The manager's role in training and staff development', in Cattermole, F., Airs, M. and Grisbrook, D. (eds) *Managing Youth Services*, Harlow: Longman, pp. 63–87.

Pollert, A. (1981) *Girls, Wives, Factory Lives*, London: Macmillan.

Rigg, C. and Trehan, K. (1999) 'Not critical enough? Black women raise challenges for critical management learning', *Gender and Education*, 11(3): 265–80.

Schein, E. H. (1965) *Organisational Psychology*, Boston: Allyn and Bacon.

Sugar, A. (2005) *The Apprentice*, London: BBC Books.

Taylor, F. (1947) *Scientific Management*, London: Harper and Row.

Twelvetrees, A. (1987) 'Accountable for change', in Cattermole, F., Airs, M. and Grisbrook, D. (eds) *Managing Youth Services*, Harlow: Longman, pp. 50–62.

Young, K. (2005) *The Art of Youth Work* (2nd edn) Lyme Regis: RHP.

# 5 Are youth work leaders free to lead?

## An exploration of the policy constraints

*Sue Lea*

This chapter sets out to critically evaluate leadership in youth work. It argues that an understanding of leadership must be grounded in an appreciation of the complex interactions between practice and broader neoliberal policy agendas. As well as drawing on the policy framework for youth work, this chapter also explores the related policy landscapes of early years and formal education. It examines the demands and constraints of a policy agenda which is driving change in both youth work and a wider range of approaches to the education and welfare of young people and children. The chapter will argue that policy interventions extend their reach through performance management, target setting, national qualification and curriculum frameworks as well as through the mechanisms of Ofsted inspection regimes. It is further argued that this policy climate severely limits the capacity of leaders to lead, and on the contrary, leaders are becoming mere conduits for national policy directives. This raises fundamental questions about the implications of an uncritical acceptance of current leadership discourses and concludes by suggesting an alternative 'democratic' approach to leadership must be built across professional boundaries.

Appropriate forms of leadership for youth work rest on beliefs and values about the nature and purpose of the work we do, and these do not exist in isolation of political, social and economic contexts in which practice is located. This chapter explores how neoliberal policy discourses aimed at surveillance and control of educational engagements are positioning the role of leaders in a changing service environment which transforms youth work, education, employment and training from a right to a duty evidenced by the objectification of young people who are not in employment, education or training (NEETs). The chapter goes on to draw on evidence from targeted interventions in the early years and in schools, concluding that not only should the dominant discourse of a particular type of transformational leadership be challenged but that this is best done by establishing networks across related professions.

### Theories of leadership

Leadership is a complex and contested concept with multiple dimensions and no clear definition (Northouse 2010). Mullins suggests there are over 400 definitions of leadership which present a minefield through which practitioners and theorists must tread (1999: 253). Theories of leadership can be viewed from a variety of perspectives and originally emerged from within a tradition which explored the actions of 'great men', often military leaders (Northouse 2010). These 'trait' theories of leadership argued that leaders are 'born' and that leadership is a personal quality which cannot be taught or learned, although arguably trait theories have been superseded and the view of leadership based upon inherent qualities has been challenged. For example, according to Handy (1993, cited in Cole 2004), by 1950 over 100 studies had taken place and only 5 per cent of the traits were common across the studies. Northouse argues, however, that trait approaches have not disappeared but have been adapted and refined and they continue to inform leadership and research. This is typified by the current emphasis in England on the role of the visionary and 'heroic' headteacher who is needed to turn around a failing school. While more recent work on emotional intelligence supports the notion that personal and social competencies are important in leadership, Goleman (2004) suggests these personal qualities can be acquired and developed.

Skills theories have to some extent superseded leadership theories based upon traits. For example, research funded by the US Army explored what skills and competencies effective leaders actually needed to solve problems in organizations (see Mumford et al. in Northouse 2010). This 'skills' approach to leadership begins to identify the necessary skills within a competency-based approach to leadership. It also provides a framework for leadership development and recognizes that different skills may be appropriate at different levels within organizations. The approach therefore indicates that leadership can be taught and learned, and that effective leadership is the ability to deploy skills in appropriate circumstances. A skills approach offers the potential for a developmental approach to leadership which acknowledges that different levels of leadership exist. For example: the skills required to lead in youth work sessions differ from those required to lead a centre, or a youth service.

The move from 'trait' theories of leadership to 'style' approaches to leadership decentres the leader as an individual and focuses instead on how leaders *behave* in relation to both task and relationships to develop their own leadership style (Cole 2004). Blake and Mouton's 'leadership grid' (in Northouse 2010: 74) offers a useful conceptual map and evaluative tool to understand different leadership styles. Style approaches largely assume a linear and technocratic approach to leadership in which top-down leaders impact on 'followers', and this raises possible value contradictions for empowering approaches to practice which are often central to the approach of youth workers. It is, however, noteworthy that research is unable to establish a definitive 'best' style (ibid.), as the appropriate style is contingent on the situation.

'Situational' theories of leadership have subsequently been developed and refined in order to take into account the need to balance directive, supportive and more democratic styles of leadership, in different organizational settings (see Likert 1961, and Tannenbaum and Schmidt 1957, cited in Cole 2004: 55). These approaches to leadership, in an attempt to balance organizational objectives and the changing needs of 'subordinates', did begin to question the traditional authority of the leader and to 'democratize' the leadership process. Situational theories are often used in leadership development programmes for aspiring leaders in the private sector. According to Northouse (2010) there is limited evidence that this approach meets the needs of followers. Once again the language, power and values implied by writers on situational theories raise issues about the underlying assumptions about the meaning and purpose of leadership. Organizational needs may be given priority and inevitably decentre the importance of professional practitioners and young people in youth work settings.

Leadership theory has acquired a more diverse and contextual approach in recent years. In a youth work context, Ford et al. (2005) note that the complexity of the leadership challenge in modern service and policy environments has led to prioritization of a 'transformational' approach to leadership. This relies on vision, consent and commitment rather than 'control and sanctions' (Ford et al. 2005: 84). Superficially this starts to move theories of leadership towards a more appropriate value framework for leading in youth work settings. However, further analysis reveals that there is almost an explicit undermining of the 'professional self' within transformational leadership as opposed to its predecessor, transactional leadership.

Harrison et al. note that transactional leadership places the practitioner centrally within the leadership process. For example transactional leadership 'recognises what it is that we want to get from work [and] … is responsive to our immediate self interests' (2007: 13). On the contrary, transformational leadership has the intention of almost overriding practitioners' own interests, as transformational leadership: 'raises our level of awareness, our level of consciousness about the significance and value of designated outcomes … gets us to transcend our own self-interest, for the sake of the team, organization or larger polity' (ibid.). Transformational leadership is therefore consistent with the neoliberal assault on professional integrity. This raises questions about the complex issues of accountability between practitioners, young people and the wider community in youth work. Leadership in youth work must reflect youth work values and practices. This is acknowledged by Ford et al., who claim that 'in some respects youth work management has characteristics which are unique to managing youth work' (2005: 14). However, they acknowledge that in this area 'there is a general absence of literature and thought' (ibid.). This chapter is designed to contribute to a 'discussion' about what appropriate forms of leadership for youth work might be.

## Neoliberal discourse and 'transformational' leadership

Despite multiple definitions and theories of leadership, it is arguably at its very least 'a relationship through which one person influences the behavior or actions of other people' (Mullins 1999: 253). However, important questions remain about the values and purposes underlying leadership and whether or not discourses are being constructed for emancipation or domestication. In order to answer this question we must critically explore the ways in which policy imposes specific demands and constraints on leaders and limits their choices. If we approach leadership with this central question in mind it becomes necessary to challenge dominant discourses and to raise questions about whether or not leaders are free to lead practice which is consistent with youth work values, or if their role is merely to implement centrally determined policy directives.

As leaders become enmeshed in the complex realities of managing change, restructuring organizations and potentially creating new professional identities, two further ethical questions emerge:

> Are youth workers (as well as other leaders in children's services) accountable to their organizations and employers or to the children and young people whose interests they claim to serve;
> To what extent should professional workers be constrained and directed by leaders in their organizations.

> (McCulloch and Tett 2010)

Since the late 1990s the dominant leadership discourse has been one of transformational leadership. This concept, however, needs to be contested, as it is a good example of 'putting words to work' (see Chapter 2). The notion of transformation being promoted is not consistent with what is meant by transformation for many youth work professionals, which is most often interpreted as the positive transformation of the lives of marginalized and oppressed young people. This raises key questions about '*who* is to determine whether the new directions are good and more affirming? *Who* decides that a new vision is a better vision?' (Northouse 2010: 189, original emphasis). Dahlberg and Moss (2005) use Foucault's work to demonstrate how power operates to create discourses and dominant regimes of truth which obscure the assumptions and values embedded in them. They highlight how power can operate through regimes of truth through which 'the ethical and political are transformed into the technical and managerial' (2005: 142) as is the case with the notion of transformational leadership.

The real danger of an uncritical acceptance of current managerial interventions and leadership discourses, is that in the name of a *particular interpretation of transformation*, it will deliver integrated policies which aim to normalize (children and) young people. Quite literally there may be no escape from the neoliberal, market-driven rationality embedded across all aspects of educational engagements (Bansel 2007). This particular interpretation of leadership is now a crucial thread which is being woven into the policy fabric of educational interventions and into the lives of children and young people (Lea 2010). Quite simply, whilst appearing to be neutral and natural, an uncritical acceptance of the practice of 'transformational' leadership has the capacity to create a service environment where children's and young people's interests are sacrificed to the technical and managerial needs of the market system. This process frames children and young people primarily as economic agents, as is evidenced in the objectification of young people as NEETs.

## Leadership in youth work contexts

Jeffs and Smith referred to the climate of neoliberalism in youth work as a 'new authoritarianism' where, 'profoundly reactionary policies are often clothed in radical and progressive rhetoric which has enabled anti-democratic practice and a controlling ideology to become embedded in the discourse of youth policy and practice' (1994: 29). It is argued, however, that it was not until the arrival of New Labour that the neoliberal reforms really began to bite. First, the arrival of Connexions (DfES 2000; 2001) began to formally construct youth work into a targeted service by emphasizing work directed at young people not in employment, education or training (NEETs). Second, the arrival of Transforming Youth Work (DfES 2001; 2002) made significant changes to the leadership, management and delivery of youth work through the introduction of managerialist performance targets. Transforming Youth Work placed a significant emphasis on leadership and management, quite clearly setting out: 'what government expects a local authority to provide through its strategic leadership role' (DfES 2002: 4) (see Chapter 2 for more details on the neoliberal policy context in youth work). Importantly this role was integrally linked to the delivery of prespecified policy priorities. For example, it was made quite clear that the youth service should: 'Provide strategic leadership for the whole service; ensure the local authority youth service is a key contributing partner to the Connexions service and local preventative strategies' (DfES 2002: 9). The importance of leadership and management was also evident when they became one of the four themes of OFSTED inspections. This parallels the managerialist ideology introduced into formal education.

Subsequent policies, ECM (DfES 2002) and Youth Matters (DfES 2005; 2006), precipitated a move away from direct local government provision, towards purchaser–provider splits with an emphasis on commissioning and the introduction of competition (Davies 2008: 48–50). The demands and constraints imposed on leaders in respect of these policies were cemented by a performance culture where top-down accountabilities aimed to ensure the leader's compliance with policy objectives through inspection and audit regimes. As a result, leaders were required to comply with centrally driven demands which targeted particular groups for surveillance and intervention, while the compliance of those leaders was also subject to similar surveillance and judgement. De St Croix notes that this 'surveillance puts the control of youth work outside the site of practice' (2010: 149). Effectively this moved the accountability of organizations, leaders, and youth workers away from young people and towards the policy demands of the neoliberal state.

Shaw (2006) highlights the problem of challenging discourses which often obscure the politics embedded in the resulting practice, a situation where we end up 'talking left and walking right'. At the heart of the contradiction is the issue of power. Despite policy makers utilizing the rhetoric of empowering leaders and/or empowering young people, they may mean very different things to what front-line professionals mean. The notion of empowerment becomes part of a discourse which gives the appearance of changing power relations while nothing actually changes at all. Similarly, leadership appears as part of a discourse of freedom and transformation, while performance indicators and inspectorates place demands and constraints on the leader which define leadership within specific parameters. The notion of choice regarding the direction of transformative change is effectively curtailed and rendered useless when transformation is limited to the leader's implementation of a top-down neoliberal policy agenda.

## Leadership and the policy panopticon

These changes are not specific to youth work, and as previously alluded to they are consistent across other educational domains including early years, schools and post-compulsory, and higher education. The neoliberal state is now directly involved (or indirectly through quangos), in the specification of curriculum from birth to 19; the education and training of professionals who work with children and young people; and leadership development. This span of control applies to leaders within formal, informal and non-formal education who are effectively constrained by the operation of 'policy technologies including choice, performance management and competition' (Ball 2008: 13). Policy compliance is further being driven by centralized forms of leadership development via the National College for School Leadership and Children's Services (NCSL) and the Children's Workforce Development Council (CWDC), where leadership discourses which appear to be neutral actually rest on the active construction of a particular interpretation of the need for reform.

Leadership is given central importance in the process of achieving policy compliance, as evidenced by moves to develop common approaches to leadership development. CWDC commissioned a report for their children's service leadership programme which reported that children's workforce development 'is a formidable challenge' (Hartle et al.

2008). 'It will require a massive culture change for most practitioners and this will happen only if there are significant shifts in the way managers, at all levels, behave [and that] having strong, skilled leaders and managers has been identified as being a significant factor' (2008: 9). The National College of School Leadership had already previously concluded that their approach to leadership development is 'to develop an "irreducible core" of management and leadership abilities ... the bedrock on which every profession must build' (Purcell 2009). Although it should be noted that leader performance becomes judged solely on the extent to which they meet centrally determined policy objectives for 'transformation' of services.

For Kanter (1981: 222) it is the focus on targets which undermines leadership in educational contexts because 'educational systems are characterized by a multiplicity, ambiguity, and diffuseness of goals ... [where] such measures come to substitute for attaining the more intangible goals of a system'. Quite simply, what counts is only that which can be measured. Gewirtz identifies these mechanisms through which criteria set by the state are now being achieved in schools, 'through the strategies of target setting, performance monitoring and closer surveillance', and highlights how the policy rhetoric of devolution is not matched by a devolution of power to leaders at the local level (Gewirtz 2002: 6).

Within early years education there is a pre-specification of curriculum with an expectation that the early years professionals demonstrate their leadership of the change agenda. The role of Ofsted has also expanded to encompass pre-school inspections alongside school and youth work inspections. The purpose of inspections is to measure performance, and with it compliance to centrally predetermined policy targets. Strategic direction was set through Children's Trusts and Children's Plans, where integrated working at the local level was supported by common assessment frameworks. Although aspects of this policy are likely to change under the coalition government, it could still be argued that the sophisticated centralized mechanisms which circumvent professionalism and bureaucratic power are already embedded. Leadership in 'the advanced liberal state, like neoliberal economics, espouses a strategy of freedom – but of a certain kind' (Dahlberg and Moss 2005: 45).

By adopting this broader framework of understanding, it is possible to develop a critical analysis of the impact of leadership. Studies of leadership in early years education is producing new ways of thinking about leadership, and like Ford et al. (2005), Rodd claims 'it is evident that the traditional themes and ideas about leadership are not really applicable to early childhood' (Rodd 2006: 10). This also reflects schools-based critiques typified by Ball (2006) and Gewirtz (2002: 49), who argue that managerialist approaches result in 'headteachers and teachers find[ing] themselves enmeshed in value conflicts and ethical dilemmas, as they are forced to rethink long-held commitments'. Fink further argues that in both Canada and the UK there is 'government pressure on school leaders to make a flawed system work ... and achieve more in a climate of politically biased, systemic, cleverly orchestrated criticism and humiliation' (2005: 9). It is clear that questions about the nature and purpose of leadership are now being raised across the educational domain, and these are relevant to youth work.

Youth work is now becoming a part of a policy panopticon being created around children and young people aged 0–19. Policy technologies now measure, count and evaluate the progress of children against socially constructed norms of development throughout their formative years in order to design interventions aimed at normalizing children and young people. The purpose of these interventions must be called into question as leadership, education and youth work are now being woven together within policy discourses where education 'is now the centre of economic policy making for the future [and where] complaining about globalization is as pointless as trying to turn back the tide' (Blair 2006, in Ball 2008: 14). Not only does the correlation between education and the labour market need to be called into question, but so does the rationality of the global neoliberal marketplace which sees education, both formal and informal, purely as a mechanism for normalizing interventions into the lives of children and young people (Bansel 2007).

## Reclaiming leadership

A key challenge to leaders in youth work and other educational settings is therefore to deconstruct *both* the policy and the leadership discourses operating in services for children and young people. By doing this we can begin to understand their combined potential to circumvent professionalism and local accountability (see Ball 2008: 13). As has been argued, if leadership is explored without reference to broader policy developments then it can appear to be neutral but, if as Ball (ibid.) argues, we understand the force and impact of policy technologies which are based on the active construction of the need for both educational and leadership reform, we can then begin to understand how the economic roles of education and youth work have become intertwined with economic and market rationalities.

The struggle over ideas is always located within discourse, and as informal educators we need to recognize that discourse has 'the performative power to bring into being the very realities it claims to describe' (Bourdieu and Wacquant 2001, in Fairclough 2001: 6). We therefore need to take Ball's claim seriously, that policy technologies are mechanisms for reforming teachers – 'changing what it means to be a teacher' – and that this highlights the real threat to practice. The analysis equally applies to youth workers and leaders, as within the reform agenda 'there are embedded and required new identities, new forms of interaction and new values', and with that comes the creation of new subjectivities (Ball 2003: 217).

If youth work is to produce truly transformational leaders, the need for critically reflective debates about the meaning and purpose of leadership in youth work will be of key importance. One helpful approach might be the 7C model of social change which identifies 'collaboration, consciousness of self, commitment, congruence, common purpose, controversy, with civility and citizenship' (Astin and Astin 2000, in Kezar and Carducci 2009: 23). Post-modern leadership paradigms now offer critical insights into leadership which are focused on leading in genuinely participatory and empowering ways and are characterized by mutual power and influence. Collective processes are indicated which question the norms and values on which existing leadership practice rests. These approaches therefore require a parallel deconstruction of traditional leadership discourses which assume existing power relations, and a reconstruction of what it means to lead 'genuine' transformative change. Such a reconstruction would need to account for youth work values which challenge existing exclusions arising from poverty and social class, as well as sexism, racism, homophobia, disablism and ageism. In summary, we need to consider the ways in which leadership in youth work might generate more inclusive, holistic, and democratic practices.

## Reconstructing youth work leadership

Within youth work we need to deconstruct neoliberal policy-driven leadership discourses and reconstruct leadership for education as a social good (Sandel 2010) and as a value-explicit, collective practice. This task sits beyond prescription and is located in democratic education and conversation. Here practice starts with relationships and the 'purposeful process of experience, reflection and learning' (Young 1999: 5) which aims to examine values, deliberate on moral judgements, and make informed decisions about choices, which lead to actions. Leaders in youth work *need* to return to the notion of educational conversations – *we must practise what we preach*.

Globalization has resulted in an increase in complexity in which older, scientific ideas of leadership are rapidly becoming obsolete where 'leadership assumptions often focus on data and strategy rather than values and beliefs' (Kezar 2009: 19). Kezar and Carducci (2009: 5) suggest that new leadership paradigms which emphasize 'interdependence, awareness of cultural and social differences, and adaptability' are now needed. They claim leadership is a process and not a possession, that culture and context matter; they call for leadership as a collaborative and collective process, the importance of mutual power and influence, and for a leadership concerned with learning, empowerment and change (ibid.: 6). This is a real challenge for education and welfare professionals where distinctive vocational cultures and values have emerged *because of* a need to negotiate the demands of working both 'in and against' the state. Collaboration between In Defence of Youth Work (IDYW 2011) and Social Work Action Network (SWAN 2011) opens up new possibilities for building cross-border alliances from which a new values-driven leadership paradigm might yet emerge. If leaders in youth work, and broader services for children and young people, fail to articulate alternative values and visions for their work, they not only lose the right to call themselves leaders, but more importantly they potentially undermine the rights of workers, children and young people in favour of neoliberal governmentalities.

Davies (2010) claims that ultimately policy is dependent in practice on what workers do, their values, intentions and methods. The 'transformational' leader of youth work needs to locate their practice at the intersection between top-down policy and organizational requirements, in the local innovative spaces which support the relationships between youth workers and young people, and in the matrix of professional interventions which are increasingly constituting and reconstituting young people's lives. It is through the language of complexity that it may be possible 'to see the non-linear, unpredictable and generative character of educational processes and practices in a positive light, focusing on the emergence of meaning, knowledge, understanding, the world and the self in and through education' (Biesta and Osberg 2010: 2). This is a key leadership challenge for youth work.

If leadership of youth work (and related services for children and young people) is to have any meaning and purpose beyond the implementation of policy, leaders will need to build alternative visions of both present and future service delivery *with* both children and young people, and with other professionals. This is both a democratic and educational endeavour and must rest on a conversation which recognizes the rights of the child (Baxter and Frederickson 2005: 99). This will require that leaders recognize their own agency and challenge the notion that they are mere conduits for the inter-related policy technologies of 'the market, managerialism and performativity' identified by Ball (2003: 215).

## *Collaboration*

As we have seen, the analysis of leadership extends beyond youth work to encompass a number of other educational (and welfare) domains. As a result, arguably, youth workers will need to reformulate their own notions of genuinely transformative leadership as they develop collective forms of cross-border reflections, conversations and professional alliances which could be built around a shared understanding of the needs and rights of children and young people (Baxter and Frederickson 2005: 99). Coburn's (2010) call for 'border crossing' to create alternative forms of knowledge, and Batsleer's call for youth workers to 'locate their story in a broader set of stories about education' (2010: 162) represent the early stages of this process.

Educational researchers have started to expose the extent to which global neoliberal agendas have extended their surveillance and control of educational engagements and relationships (Apple 2001; 2005; Smith 2002; Biesta 2006; Bansel 2007; Lea 2010). Like Coburn (2010) and Batsleer (2010), Dahlberg and Moss (2005) also call for analytical 'border-crossing' and highlight the need to deconstruct the formation of pedagogical relationships, and relations of power and knowledge which span the educational domain from pre-school to higher education. They stress the need for new discourses which challenge the pervasive tendency towards the normalization of children and young people, while leadership discourses move in opposition.

There are some signs of dissent within professional groupings: for example, the development of the In Defence of Youth Work campaign (IDYW 2011) and the Social Work Action Network (SWAN 2011). In order to reclaim youth work and its leadership role from neoliberal educational policy, alliances will need to be built across professional boundaries which include both practitioners and researchers. In Defence of Youth Work and the Social Work Action Network held a joint conference in January 2011, which indicates this may already be happening.

## Conclusion

Perhaps with the move to the 'big society' (see Chapter 13) and the partial dismantling of the managerialist state resulting from the unprecedented public sector cuts, a space may be created within which to develop a debate about more democratic forms of leadership. Indeed, the Local Government Association (LGA 2010: 3) has recently argued for strong local leadership with accountability to the electorate rather than government inspectors, and has called for the liberation of local service provision from 'unnecessary controls'.

It is nearly a century since Dewey wrote that a 'democracy is more than a form of government; it is primarily a mode of associated living, of conjoint communicated experience' (Dewey 1916: 87). Democracy, particularly local democracy, is an essential precondition for leaders who wish to empower young people and deliver highly responsive, inclusive educational opportunities. It is high time that leadership returned democracy to centre stage.

## Questions for reflection and discussion

1    What are the key similarities and differences between locality-based and centralized visions, for the transformation of youth work?

2    How can we judge if a new leader's vision for youth work is a better vision than the one which currently exists?
3    What might be the core values of a leader who you would be most likely to follow? To what extent are leaders in services for children and young people merely the conduits for compliance with central policy objectives?

## Further reading

Batsleer, J. and Davies, B. (eds) (2010) *What Is Youth Work?* Exeter: Learning Matters.
Fink, D. (2005) *Leadership for Mortals: Developing and Sustaining Leaders of Learning*, London: Paul Chapman Publishing.
Kezar, A. (ed.) (2009) *Rethinking Leadership in a Complex Multicultural and Global Environment*, Sterling, VA: Stylus.
Rodd, J. (2006) *Leadership in Early Childhood* (3rd edn) Maidenhead: Open University Press.

## References

Apple, M. W. (2005) 'Doing things the "right" way: legitimating educational inequalities in conservative times', *Educational Review*, 57: 271–93.
——(2001) 'Comparing the neoliberal project and inequality in education', *Comparative Education*, 37(4): 409–23.
Ball, S. J. (2008) *The Education Debate*, Bristol: Policy Press.
——(2006) *Education Policy and Social Class: The Selected Works of Stephen J. Ball*, London: Routledge.
——(2003) 'The teachers' soul and the terrors of performativity', *Journal of Education Policy*, 18 (2): 215–28.
Banks, S. (ed.) (1999) *Ethical Issues in Youth Work*, London: Routledge.
Bansel, P. (2007) 'Subject of choice and lifelong learning', *International Journal of Qualitative Studies in Education*, 20(3): 283–300.
Barker, R. (ed.) (2009) *Making Sense of Every Child Matters: Multi-professional Guidance*, Bristol: Policy Press.
Batsleer, J. (2010) 'Youth work prospects: back to the future?', in Batsleer, J. and Davies, B. (eds) *What Is Youth Work?* Exeter: Learning Matters, pp. 153–65.
Batsleer, J. and Davies, B. (eds) (2010) *What Is Youth Work?* Exeter: Learning Matters.
Baxter, J. and Frederickson, N. (2005) 'Every Child Matters: can educational psychology contribute to radical reform?', *Educational Psychology in Practice*, 21(2): 87–102.
Biesta, G. (2006) 'What's the point of lifelong learning if lifelong learning has no point? On the democratic deficit of policies for lifelong learning', *European Educational Research Journal*, 3(3): 169–80.
Biesta, G. and Osberg, D. (2010) 'Complexity, education and politics from the inside-out and the outside-in', in Osberg, D. and Biesta, G. (eds) *Complexity Theory and the Politics of Education*, Rotterdam: Sense, pp. 1–5.
Bourdieu, P. and Wacquant, L. J. D. (1992) *An Invitation to Reflexive Sociology*, Cambridge: Polity Press.
Coburn, A. (2010) 'Youth work as border pedagogy', in Batsleer, J. and Davies, B. (eds) *What Is Youth Work?* Exeter: Learning Matters, pp. 33–46.
Cole, G. A. (2004) *Management Theory and Practice* (6th edn) London: Thomson.
Dahlberg, G. and Moss, P. (2005) *Ethics and Politics in Early Childhood Education*, London: RoutledgeFalmer.
Davies, B. (2008) *The New Labour Years: A History of the Youth Service in England, Volume 3*, Leicester: Youth Work Press.

——(2010) 'What do we mean by youth work?', in Batsleer, J. and Davies, B. (eds) *What Is Youth Work?* Exeter: Learning Matters, pp. 1–6.

De St Croix, T. (2010) 'Youth work and the surveillance state', in Batsleer, J. and Davies, B. (eds) *What Is Youth Work*? Exeter: Learning Matters, pp. 140–52.

Dewey, J. (1916) *Democracy and Education: An Introduction to the Philosophy of Education*, New York: The Free Press.

DfCSF (2010) 'Aiming Higher for Young People': Three Years on, www.education.gov.uk/publications/eOrderingDownload/00331-2010DOM-EN.pdf (accessed 2 May 2010).

DfES (2006) *Youth Matters – The Next Steps*, London: HMSO.

——(2005) *Youth Matters*, London: HMSO.

——(2003) *Every Child Matters*, London: HMSO.

——(2002) *Transforming Youth Work: Resourcing Excellent Youth Services*, London: HMSO.

——(2001) *Understanding Connexions*, London HMSO.

——(2000) *Connexions: The Best Start in Life for Every Young Person*, www.lga.gov.uk/lga/parliament/connexions.pdf

Drucker, P. F. (2002) *Management Challenges for the 21st Century*, Oxford: Elsevier Butterworth-Heinemann.

Fairclough, N. (2001) *The Dialectics of Discourse*, www.ling.lancs.ac.uk/profiles/263 (accessed 30 July 2009.

Fink, D. (2005) *Leadership for Mortals: Developing and Sustaining Leaders of Learning*, London: Paul Chapman Publishing

Ford, K., Hunter, R., Merton, B. and Waller, D. (2005) *Leading and Managing Youth Work and Services for Young People*, Leicester: National Youth Agency.

Gewirtz, S. (2002) *The Managerial School: Post-welfarism and Social Justice in Education*, London: Routledge.

Goleman, D. (2004) *Emotional Intelligence and Working with Emotional Intelligence*, London: Bloomsbury.

Grint, K. (2005) 'Problems, problems, problems: the social construction of "leadership"', *Human Relations*, 58(11): 1467–94.

Harrison, R., Benjamin, C., Curran, S. and Hunter, R. (2007) *Leading Work with Young People*, London: Sage/Open University Press.

Hartle, F., Snook, P., Apsey, H. and Browton, R. (2008) *The Training and Development of Middle Managers in the Children's Workforce*, www.cwdcouncil.org.uk (retrieved 6 May 2010).

IDYW (2011), *In Defence of Youth Work*, www.indefenceofyouthwork.org.uk/wordpress/ (accessed 11 March 2011).

Jeffs, T. and Smith, M. K. (1994) 'Young people, youth work and a new authoritarianism', *Youth and Policy*, Autumn, no. 46: 17–32.

Kanter, R. M. (1981) 'Power, leadership and participatory management', *Theory into Practice*, 20 (4): 219–228.

Kezar, A. (ed.) (2009) *Rethinking Leadership in a Complex Multicultural and Global Environment*, Sterling, VA: Stylus.

Kezar, A. and Carducci, R. (2009) 'Revolutionizing leadership development', in Kezar, A. (ed.) *Rethinking Leadership in a Complex Multicultural and Global Environment*, Sterling, VA: Stylus, pp. 1–38.

Lea, S. (2010) 'Educational relationships, reflexivity and values in a time of global economic fundamentalism', *Critical and Reflective Practice in Education*, vol. 2: 80–91. www.marjon.ac.uk/research/criticalandreflectivepracticeineducation/volume2 (retrieved 14 December 2010).

LGA (Local Government Association) (July 2010) Report: Local Freedom or Central Control? Why Councils Have an Important Role to Play in Local Education, www.lga.gov.uk (retrieved 12 August 2010).

McCulloch, K. and Tett, L. (2010) 'Professional ethics of youth work', in Banks, S. (ed.) *Ethical Issues in Youth Work* (2nd edn) London: Routledge, pp. 38–52.

Mullins, L. (1999) *Management and Organisational Behaviour* (5th edn) Harlow: Pearson Education.

NCSL (undated) *Meeting the Need: Extract of Recommendations*, www.ncsl.org.uk (retrieved 7 September 2006).

Northouse, P. G. (2010) *Leadership: Theory and Practice* (5th edn) Thousand Oaks, CA: Sage.

Ord, J. (2007) *Youth Work: Process, Product and Practice*, Lyme Regis: Russell House Publishing.

Potter, J. (undated) *Leadership: Handling the Human Side of Complexity*, www.ifm.eng.cam.ac.uk (retrieved 1 June 2010).

Prilleltensky, I. (2000) 'Value-based leadership in organizations: balancing values, interests, and power among citizens, workers and leaders', *Ethics and Behavior*, 10(2): 139–58.

Purcell, M. (2009) 'Leadership development programme for current and aspirant directors of children's services', www.ncsl.org.uk (retrieved 5 May 2010).

Rodd, J. (2006) *Leadership in Early Childhood* (3rd edn) Maidenhead: Open University Press.

Sandel, M. (2010) 'Markets and morals: a new citizenship', Reith lectures, available at downloads. bbc.co.uk/.../20090609_thereithlectures_marketsandmorals.rtf (accessed 4 April 2011).

Shaw, M. (2006) 'Community development – everywhere and nowhere? Rediscovering the purpose and practice of community development', Conference paper to the Scottish Community Development Network, 9 March, www.scdn.org.uk (retrieved 5 November 2009).

Smith, M. K. (2002) 'Transforming youth work – Resourcing excellent youth services: a critique', The Informal Education Homepage, www.infed.org/youthwork/transforming _youth_ work_2.htm

SWAN (2011) *Social Work Action Network*, www.socialworkfuture.org/ (accessed 3 March 2011).

Young, K. (1999) *The Art of Youth Work*, Lyme Regis: Russell House Publishing.

# 6 Planning

## For opportunities not outcomes

*Jon Ord*

It is accepted that planning is an essential feature of youth work practice, in that it both helps to set direction in terms of overall strategy, as well as coordinate the decisions required for action on a day-to-day basis. Milburn (2001) reminds us of the importance of 'planning ahead' as a managerial task; however, planning in youth work is complex. Despite this there are increasingly simplistic demands on youth workers to plan their work in specific detail. It is assumed there is a specific relationship between those plans and the predicted outcomes of youth work. Furthermore youth workers are increasingly being made accountable for those pre-specified outcomes. It is this highly problematic situation which this chapter will attempt to address.

Planning is essentially 'future focused' and 'in all plans ... there will be an attempt to predict what will happen in the future' (Hannagan, 2008: 182). It could be argued that unless work is well planned one has little control over what will happen in the youth centre or project. Too little planning results in an uncertain future, and the resulting youth work practice can only be reactive, responding to what occurs in the 'here and now'. Much good youth work results from this 'reactive' approach, and this flexibility of being able to respond to what is pertinent to young people at that particular moment – 'going with the flow' (Jeffs and Smith, 2005: 33) should never be entirely lost. However:

> It is easy for a unit to drift on from week to week. That usually results in the workers and young people becoming bored, because the work is reactive and patterned. The purpose of planning is to move from being reactive to being proactive and to gain some control over your work.
>
> (Ingram and Harris, 2001: 43)

Proactive youth work is of equal importance and it is planning which enables proactive youth work to take place; in the short term thinking about issues that need to be dealt with, trying to organize the time to have those conversations that need to be had, organizing activities that young people require, etc. Planning also enables medium- and long-term projects to take place where more detailed planning is required, for example where resources need to be put in place.

One of the problems with planning, however, is predicting the future, and as working with young people in an informal setting necessarily takes place in an uncertain environment, producing both inappropriate and unreliable plans is always a possibility. On this basis the further the plan 'reaches' into the future, the less reliable that plan becomes. For example at the beginning of the term it may have appeared like a good idea to plan for an end-of-term residential with the current group of young people who attend the youth centre, but as the term progressed a number of other issues arose both within the group such as bullying, personal problems or issues at school, as well as perhaps between the existing group and a number of new arrivals involving fluctuations in relationships and group dynamics, and the workers may decide quite rightly that the needs arising from the current issues are not best met by going on a residential. So the residential becomes a long-term possibility rather than a medium-term probability. On this basis Hannagan (2008) argues that all good plans should contain 'contingencies'. Mintzberg (2000) also notes that one needs a flexible approach to planning, as both too much planning as well as too little planning can both lead to chaos. The problem with 'rigid adherence' to a plan is one loses flexibility of response, and in the 'absence of plan', one has limited control over future development, and is a 'hostage to fortune'.

## Planning in youth work

Planning is acknowledged as an essential ingredient of youth work practice (Smith, 1994; Ingram and Harris, 2001; Riley, 2001). Riley (2001) identifies the importance of an organization's 'overall aim' as a guide for youth workers in how they plan and deliver their work. The aim should, according to Riley, 'convey the ethos of youth work', but should be broad enough to enable: 'the implementation of a wide variety of learning experiences and opportunities' (2001: 148). First and foremost, according to Riley, any plan should be based on the needs of young people, but should also involve considerations of the 'timescale' and 'environment', as well as the 'constraints'. Although Riley does implicitly acknowledge Mintzberg's and Hannigan's point that planning must involve: 'flexibility ... to allow for, and encompass, deviations from intended outcomes' (2001: 149).

Riley maintains the importance of three levels of planning: Short-term activities, medium-term projects and long-term projects. She describes quizzes, discussion groups and activities as examples of short-term projects. Through the planning of these: 'the worker is able to evaluate sessions and plan future interventions around areas of concern' (2001: 150). Medium-term projects 'need more thought, preparation and planning. They can be designed to promote involvement from members and require a firm commitment before the event can take place' (2001: 151). These medium-term projects allow the worker to tailor the youth work programme to better meet the developmental needs of young people. Tasks can be allocated appropriately, support and guidance can be given where necessary, and young people gain confidence from succeeding in delivering what they had planned; whether that be a trip away, or a special event at the youth centre. Longer-term projects require greater commitment from the young people and the workers can enable greater levels of 'responsibility, leadership and organizational roles' to be taken on by young people. Riley rightly points out that youth workers ought to be able to 'let go', and with this come new problems and challenges in terms of planning. Such participative practices (Baker, 1996; Barber, 2007; Ord, 2007) should be at the heart of the planning process. But of course the extent to which any outcome can be assured is potentially undermined by the risks of 'handing over the reins' to young people.

However, some argue planning is of much less significance. Smith does recognize 'when running residentials, short courses, activity programmes ... [workers] do plan in such a [specific] way' (1994: 80). However, he argues: 'the nature of the physical and social context and character of the interactions necessitate a less prescriptive ... form of planning' (ibid.). With the emphasis on conversation, informal educators such as Smith place more emphasis on 'assessing' and 'discerning' what arises out of the interactions and dialogue than on the delivery of a preplanned educational intervention. This approach is further developed by Jeffs and Smith (2005), where little reference is made to the importance of planning. However, they do acknowledge that on occasion a preplanned approach is appropriate, for example on issues of health education. In general they argue against a planned approach, instead advocating the need for 'going with the flow'.

Ingram and Harris (2001) on the contrary give a central role to the planning process in the delivery of 'good' youth work. Their approach contrasts markedly with that of Jeffs and Smith, suggesting that planning in youth work is clearly structured and 'systematic'. They argue that the NAOMIE model underpins the planning process in youth work, which involves: identifying the *Need*, setting the *Aim* and *Objectives*, followed by the selection of a *Method*, *Implementation* and *Evaluation* (Ingram and Harris, 2001: 20). This approach is open to interpretation and can be implemented rigidly or with some flexibility, but as we shall see later there is a danger that in the current climate the more rigid application will predominate.

There is a sense in which both these approaches to planning, although different, can be problematic. Smith (1994) and Jeffs and Smith (2005) arguably give too little credence to the importance of the preplanned educational intentions of youth workers. Unless work is clearly planned, whether that be short-, medium- or long-term, it will be impoverished, in that workers are less able to be proactive in their interventions and are dependent on what emerges from the participants (Ord, 2007). Whilst the advantage of their approach is that it maximizes the responsiveness of the workers to what is pertinent to the young people, the work can at best only be reactive. Ingram and Harris on the contrary could be interpreted as giving too little credence to the flexibility and indeterminate nature of the process of youth work. Youth work becomes, with the implementation of its session plan, similar to the rolling out of a formal 'lesson'. Such a mechanistic approach to youth work does not provide an appropriate planning framework for youth. For planning in youth work to be effective it must build in considerable flexibility, and autonomy for the work to develop, and the ability of youth workers to respond appropriately and effectively to what emerges through the interactions.

## The cultural shift in youth work planning

Transforming Youth Work (DfES, 2001; 2002) created a significant cultural shift in the way that youth work is planned and delivered, particularly in the statutory sector. Whilst in the voluntary sector the shift from grants to contracts, which are tied to the delivery of specific outcomes, has also profoundly influenced how youth work is planned and delivered.

> The result of these changes is that the culture of youth work has changed. Youth work is no longer so spontaneous; planning is an absolute requirement, as is the paperwork that goes with it. Youth work is under scrutiny and in the public view more than ever before.
>
> (Ingram and Harris, 2001: 14)

Individual youth workers have increasingly lost the autonomy that underpinned their work. Youth work has become more centralized, with central government setting priorities (Smith, 2003). Transforming Youth Work clearly specified how youth work must be integrated into a structured planning framework, requesting: 'The development of plans by local authorities for their youth services ... the plans will link resources available to planned levels of provision' (DfES, 2002: 18). In addition the DfES provided guidance in the form of the Common Planning Framework to ensure that: 'the service will be underpinned by the National and local priorities and actions [as well as] targets' (2002: 34).

Importantly, youth work planning was specifically linked to 'outcomes'. Whilst it was acknowledged that youth work was informed by specific values and operated within a broad set of educational aims, it was made explicit that:

> Such broad goals need to be expressed in a set of more specific outcomes if they are to be helpful in the planning and in practice. The more clearly we can specify the ends, the better we will be able to choose the means for achieving them.
>
> (DfES, 2002: 11)

Youth workers were under pressure to identify in advance what they considered to be the needs of young people, as well as how they planned to meet them. Importantly, they would need to specify, in advance, what outcomes would be achieved in relation to those needs. Transforming Youth Work's expectation was quite explicit: 'In the light of these needs, what learning outcomes and content should normally be covered within a year's programme' (DfES, 2002: 27). It was made quite clear by policymakers: 'This approach [to youth work] can use informal but not *unstructured* learning strategies' (DfES, 2002: 35, author's emphasis). As Milburn pointed out, this created: 'a culture of development planning and evaluation of work for the measurement of performance indicators ... formalised statements of quality' (2001: 219). As has been argued, this undermined the informal processes of youth work (Smith, 2003; Davies, 2005; Ord, 2007).

In the subsequent years a plethora of planning protocols and frameworks have been produced, which has been exacerbated by the incorporation of youth work into Children's Trusts. These include the Common Planning Framework (2002), the Children and Young People's Plan (which was a requirement of the Children Act 2004), the Children and Young People's Plan (England) Regulations 2005, the Single Education Plan (2005), and the Children and Young People's Plan (England) (Amendment) Regulations 2007. Whilst most of the requirements to produce formalized plans have been relaxed, arguably the shift in the 'culture of planning' has remained.

At worst, this cultural shift has created a 'bureaucracy of planning' where workers spend more time predicting what it is that needs to be done, creating ways of delivering work which would in (theory at least) produce particular outputs, and outcomes (than actually delivering face-to-face work). All this in advance of undertaking the work, and sometimes even before young people have been met or relationships developed. A tier of planning has been created where area-wide development plans are produced as part of overall 'children and young people's plans'. Then annual plans and individual program plans are produced which fit into these centralized frameworks. Importantly, this is a top-down system within which the priorities are not set by individual youth workers who know and understand the needs and requirements of the young people they are working with. All this of course is within the context of specific targets which youth work must deliver on (see Chapter 9 for more a detailed discussion on the impact of targets).

## Theory of planning

As was suggested by Ford et al. (2005) (see Chapter 3 above), the dominant theoretical framework underpinning the management of organizations is systems theory. Organizations use this approach: 'to understand and monitor their performance. This involves identifying inputs, the process of transforming inputs into outputs, and the outcomes these can lead to' (Ford et al., 2005: 163). Importantly, Ford et al. (2005) claim that their 'performance model of management' is directly transferable to youth work[1] (see Figure 3.1, p. 34).

Within this model the inputs are described as: 'what goes into providing the service, usually the people, plant and pounds, including staff's knowledge' (Ford et al., 2005: 164). The process is described rather simplistically as: 'the variety of ways we work with young people' (ibid.). The outputs they define as: 'a measure of the activity that has taken place such as the volume of service, range of activities and levels of achievement' (ibid.). The outcomes are: 'the results our services have on the lives of young people who use them' (ibid.). It is clear that this model is wedded to managerialist principles, as an explanation is provided as to how the elements of this model are linked directly to the three Es:

> The cost of the imports give you a measure of the *economy* of the activity … the volume of the outputs divided by the cost of the inputs gives you a measure of the *efficiency* of the activity … the number and quality of the outcomes achieved tell you the *effectiveness* of your organization.
>
> (Ibid.)

Implicit within this model is that youth work and its associated learning is conceived of as a linear process (Ord, 2004a; 2004b). That is, there is an assumption that there is a direct and causal link between inputs and outputs, and the resulting outcomes, in the process of youth work. It is not being argued that youth work cannot be planned in such a linear fashion. Indeed, even Jeffs and Smith (2005) who place the least emphasis on planning, acknowledge, in some instances, that work is appropriately planned utilizing this product approach. However, it is problematic for youth work if its entire approach to both planning and the production of outcomes is conceptualized in a linear dimension.[2]

In the main the educational process of youth work is not linear. Smith alludes to this in his description of the relationship between many of the outcomes of youth work and the educational interventions of youth workers which brought them about: 'A central consideration has been the apparently incidental manner in which learning may occur in informal or "natural societal" situations' (1988: 126). In emphasizing the 'incidental' nature of outcomes he is not suggesting that they are accidental, and arrived at by chance. But importantly, the outcomes in youth work are, in the main, not directly related to specific interventions. The causal relationship between the process of youth work and its outcomes is best described as 'indirect'. This has important implications for how planning is conceptualized and implemented.

Interestingly, not only are the outcomes of youth work often incidental but paradoxically in some cases it is actually better to not focus on the outcome in order to achieve it. This is referred to as the '*paradox of process*' (Ord, 2007: 92–95). The example of confidence or self-esteem illustrates this. In the case of this important youth work outcome, not only can it '*not be directly planned for*' in a simplistic mechanistic manner, but endlessly focusing on someone's lack of confidence is liable to undermine their confidence rather than build it.

Confidence is built incidentally over time by setting surmountable challenges, offering appropriate feedback, support and praise. As confidence is built over time any genuine growth in confidence is not proportional to any one specific intervention or other. Confidence grows as a result of a process of being engaged in the kind of things that make one feel good about oneself, developing skills, widening experience and achieving tasks. Any growth in confidence might be incremental but it comes about through what Spence et al. refer to as 'small steps' which in themselves are 'almost intangible outcomes' (2006: 31). One can try and plan youth work activities which it is hoped will provide the kinds of experiences which are likely to build, rather than undermine, confidence and esteem, but that is quite a different matter.

The incidental nature of outcomes is further illustrated by Brent (2004), who uses the example of a young girl in his club. He describes how she undergoes a profound change in her demeanour as she begins to 'smile', after attending his youth club over a period of time: 'There has been no product, no target met, no plan completed, yet all the evidence points to there being a profoundly important personal outcome for Kelly' (2004: 70). It was clear that her sense of self, her esteem and confidence had grown through being a part of the club, people taking an interest in her and her life, meeting new people, developing relationships and taking part in activities. Importantly, this significant outcome for the young person (who fitted all the criteria for government targeted work, i.e. NEET, at risk of teenage pregnancy and substance abuse, etc.) had been achieved, in that her aspirations had been raised and a number of her problems alleviated. But this work was not, and it is argued could not have been, achieved through such a formal and mechanistic planning process.

Indeed, taken to its extreme there are absurd implications of a mechanistic approach to planning. If it is assumed that a causal, linear and rational relationship exists between inputs and outputs, inputs are therefore directly proportional to outputs. This would imply that the more conversations a youth worker has, the more interventions made, the greater the number of outcomes that will be achieved, likewise the more activities undertaken the better. What, of course, is missing is an appreciation of the 'quality' of the conversations or activities. The appropriateness and 'timeliness' of the interventions cannot be accounted for in a mechanistic model. What youth workers engage young people in is a 'developmental process' which involves building relationships with young people to better understand the experience of their lives and therefore intervene appropriately. In addition the activities and programmes that are delivered are specifically geared to meeting those developmental needs. This complex and highly skilled process is not captured with any degree of accuracy in the Ford et al. (2005) model, as it relies too heavily on the linear translation of inputs to outputs. As Davies (2006) makes clear when commenting on the government's emphasis on youth workers planning for young people to take part in 'positive activities':

> This is far too simplistic. Just encouraging young people into an activity for the activity's sake will not necessarily generate affirming or positively developmental social experiences. Watch some young men on a football field berate 'a mate' whose final pass isn't inch perfect. Follow the politics of some theatre productions as the time comes to allocate parts. Where here in pursuit of 'positive activity' is a guaranteed focus on – even concern for – nurturing participants' personal

confidence, self esteem and social competence: Indeed where are the facilitation skills often vital to getting to these personally developmental outcomes?

(Davies, 2005)

## The complexity of systems theory

This critique of a mechanistic and 'technical rational' approach to planning is supported from within wider management literature and supports the questioning of the suitability of a simplistic approach to the planning of youth work. We saw that Ford et al. (2005) argue that most organizations use a systems approach, implying that all organizations utilize a similar mechanistic analogy of the translation of inputs to outputs. However, there are subtleties and complexities within systems theory itself which undermine this claim. For example Wild (1989) distinguishes between four types of organization: *manufacturer*, which involves making something; *transport*, which involves moving something or someone; *supply*, which involves providing some physical goods; and *service*, where something happens to someone or something. Importantly, he suggests that there are distinct differences in how inputs and outputs are conceived of depending on the type of organization.

If youth work is to be considered in terms of systems theory, it is on the basis that it is part of the 'service' sector. Importantly, Schmenner (1986) suggests, for organizations which are primarily 'service producers' of which he includes educational institutions, 'any tangible goods provided in connection with the service is incidental' (cited in Hannagan, 2008: 466). Johnson and Clark furthermore suggest: 'for many services, there is no clear boundary between experience and the outcome ... the education and the educational experience ... are inseparable' (2005: 13).

Schmenner (1986; 1995) goes on to suggest a number of factors associated with 'services' that make them distinct from other types of 'production' and therefore need to be managed differently. These include, first, identifying the service outputs as '*intangible*': 'services are not a thing that is produced but an activity that is experienced in some way ... the physical output from the process therefore does not exist in a tangible state' (cited in Hannagan, 2008: 467). Second, services often involve '*variable, non-standard output*', that is each example of the service is different and unique. As a result 'quality is difficult to predict' (cited in Hannagan, 2008: 468). Third, a service is often '*perishable*'. As Hannigan comments: 'A service is consumed instantly ... and cannot be stored although consumers may enjoy the benefit for a long while afterwards' (2008: 467).

Schmenner also identifies what he calls '*customer participation*' and that 'the relationship between the organization and the customer ... is a crucial factor in determination of quality' (cited in Hannagan, 2008: 468). Clearly a direct parallel, in this respect, is the involvement of young people in youth work, and the relationships that develop, which are both essential to the quality of youth work practice, but contain inherent risks in terms of enabling workers both to predict outcomes, as well as ensuring the validity of their plans. Schmenner goes on to suggest some services also involve: '*high personal judgment used by employees*'. This is another important factor implying that services cannot be mass produced, are labour-intensive and difficult to quantify. Finally, and equally relevant to planning in youth work, is Schmenner's point that for the service sector 'demand varies greatly over a short period'. Clearly as a result of this condition flexibility of planning and response is essential.

What is clearly evident is that systems theory is far from simple. The complexities of each organization need to be taken into account, as does the unique environment of each particular system. On this basis therefore, youth work and how it is planned must reflect essential elements of youth work practice rather than have an external, simplistic and linear framework superimposed upon it. It would appear that the performance model of management and the resulting simplistic expectations on youth workers to plan their work according to the prediction of pre-specified outcomes and outputs, fit neither theory nor practice. Arguably it is nothing more than a managerial tool to control youth workers, and it does little to develop or enhance youth work practice.

## A coherent approach to youth work planning

An important distinction central to the understanding of the planning process in youth work is between broad goals or aims on the one hand and specific goals or objectives on the other. Citing Brookfield (1983: 15), Smith reminds us that 'purpose and intent may not always be marked by closely specified goals' (1988: 128). That is, just because youth workers may not have, or been able to, set specific goals or objectives in the planning of their work does not mean that it lacks educational intent. At the heart of the 'problem' of planning for youth work is the extent to which it is increasingly being expected to plan by specific, rather than broad goals. The emphasis on specific goals or outcomes, rather than broad aims or goals undermines youth work's fundamental educational purpose.

There also are parallel processes present in youth work which affect how the work is planned. On the one hand is the ongoing work with individuals and groups of young people over time, based on an understanding of the young people involved. This understanding, which enables an appreciation of the needs of young people, is derived from the development of trusting relationships which are at the heart of the youth work process (Davies, 2005; Young, 2005; Ord, 2007). This work is structured in the sense that workers are aware of issues that need to be followed up on, concerns that need raising, support that needs to be offered and challenges that need to be provided. Activities need to be facilitated which enable such needs to be addressed rather than precluded. For example, if a worker is aware that a core group from the youth project needs time to reflect upon a crucial decision (for example leaving school), or an individual has an issue they want to get off their chest, space needs to be found to enable a discussion about these issues to take place. Therefore planning an evening walk or a campfire would be more conducive than a sporting activity.

At the other end of the planning process is the specific 'short-term' planned work that youth workers undertake, for example to raise awareness of sexually transmitted diseases, the dangers of smoking or of drinking too much. These are important aspects of a planned youth work programme. However, they do not and more importantly must not override the more fundamental ongoing youth work processes. Another aspect of the youth work process which in many instances produces significant outcomes for young people are the interventions made 'on the wing' – outcomes which arise from the dynamics of a particular situation which could not have been predicted, as Williamson reminds us:

> No self-respecting youth worker would wish to make the case for unstructured youth work ... [however,] structured youth work has many meanings. It is not just

about organized activities and explicitly outlined programmes of intervention [but involves] milking the learning opportunities from often unexpected and sometimes apparently disorganized moments.

(2005: 15)

Finally of course there is the problem that many of the outcomes of youth work, because of its developmental nature, become apparent weeks, months or even years 'down the line'.

To conclude, as an in-depth appreciation of systems theory makes clear (Schmenner, 1986; Johnson and Clark, 2005) any application of the theory of planning must take account of the unique circumstances of the organizational setting. The relationship between inputs and both outputs and outcomes, is unique in youth work and, it has been argued, in the main this makes planning for specific outcomes untenable. Outcomes emerge out of a process of engagement with young people. The youth work process takes place over time, and involves the deepening of relationships, the understanding of the young people concerned, and the needs that emerge out of this understanding. In this sense, therefore, it makes more sense to plan for *opportunities and not outcomes*. Youth work can still be accountable for its outcomes but it should not necessarily be able to predict with any degree of certainty what those outcomes may, or may not, be until the process of youth work has developed, and the work 'unfolded'.

## Questions for reflection and discussion

1   How can youth workers plan their work to best enable the process of youth work to develop?
2   What might be some of the differences between how youth workers plan for opportunities as opposed to planning for outcomes?
3   Given the difficulties of predicting the outcomes of youth work, how and by what means should youth workers be accountable?

## Notes

1   This was not just a theoretical exercise. 'Ford Management Partnership' delivered a large-scale training programme for youth work managers, funded by the DfES, as part of the Transforming Youth Work Development Programme agenda in 2003/4 and 2004/5.
2   This linear/product approach to the planning and delivery was further emphasized when Wiley and Merton (2002) and the DfES (2002) attempted to introduce a 'set' youth work curriculum based upon content, the pedagogy of educational group work and assessment (see Ord, 2004a; 2004b).

## Further reading

Davies, B. (2005) 'Youth work: a manifesto for our times', *Youth and Policy*, Summer, no. 88: 5–27.
Jeffs, T. and Smith, M. K. (2008) 'Valuing youth work', *Youth and Policy*, Summer/Autumn, no. 100: 227–301.
Ord, J. (2007) *Youth Work Process, Product and Practice: Creating an Authentic Curriculum in Work with Young People*, Lyme Regis: RHP.

# References

Baker, J. (1996) *The Fourth Partner: Participant or Consumer*, Leicester: Youth Work Press.

Barber, T. (2007) 'Young people and civic participation: a conceptual review', *Youth and Policy*, Summer, no. 96: 19–39.

Brent, J. (2004) 'Communicating what youth work achieves: the smile and the arch', *Youth and Policy*, Summer, no. 84: 69–73.

Davies, B. (2005) 'Youth work: a manifesto for our times', *Youth and Policy*, Summer, no. 88: 5–27.

——(2006) 'Takes issue with … Freedom's Orphans', *The Edge*, Leicester: NYA, August.

——(2008) *The New Labour Years: A History of the Youth Service in England, Volume 3, 1997 – 2007*, Leicester: NYA.

DfES (2001) *Transforming Youth Work: Developing Youth Work for Young People*, Nottingham: HMSO.

——(2002) *Transforming Youth Work: Resourcing Excellent Youth Services*, Nottingham: HMSO.

Ford, K., Hunter, R., Merton, B. and Waller, D. (2005) *Leading and Managing Youth Work and Services for Young People*, Leicester: NYA.

Hannagan, T. (2008) *Management Concepts and Practices* (5th edn) Harlow: FT/Prentice Hall.

Ingram, G. and Harris, J. (2001) *Delivering Good Youth Work*, Lyme Regis: RHP.

Jeffs, T. and Smith, M. K. (2005) *Informal Education, Conversation, Democracy and Learning* (3rd edn) Derby: Education Now.

Johnson, K. and Clark, G. (2005) *Service Operations Management, Improving Service Delivery*, Harlow: Pearson Education.

Merton, B. and Wylie, T. (2002) *Towards a Contemporary Youth Work Curriculum*, Leicester: NYA.

Milburn, T. (2001) 'Managing Work', in Deer Richardson, L. and Wolfe, M. (eds) *Principles and Practice of Informal Education*, London: RoutledgeFalmer, pp. 212–21.

Mintzberg, H. (2000) *The Rise and Fall of Strategic Planning*, Harlow: FT/Prentice Hall.

Ord, J. (2004a) 'The Youth Work Curriculum and the Transforming Youth Work Agenda', *Youth and Policy*, Spring, no. 83: 43–59.

——(2004b) 'The Youth Work Curriculum as process not as output and outcome to aid accountability', *Youth and Policy*, Autumn, no. 85: 53–69.

——(2007) *Youth Work Process, Product and Practice: Creating an Authentic Curriculum in Work with Young People*, Lyme Regis: RHP.

Riley, P. (2001) 'Programme planning', in Deer Richardson, L. and Wolfe, M. (eds) *Principles and Practice of Informal Education*, London: RoutledgeFalmer, pp. 148–57.

Schmenner, R. W. (1986) 'How can service businesses survive and prosper?' *Sloan Management Review*, Spring: 21–32.

——(1995) *Service Operations Management*, Atlantic Highlands, NJ: Prentice Hall.

Smith, M. K. (1988) *Developing Youth Work*, Milton Keynes: Open University Press.

——(1994) *Local Education: Community, Conversation, Praxis*, Buckingham: Open University Press.

——(2003) 'From youth work to youth development', *Youth and Policy*, Spring, no. 79: 46–59.

Spence, J. and Devanney, C., with Noonan, K. (2006) *Youth Work: Voices of Practice*, Leicester: NYA.

Wild, R. (1989) *Production and Operations Management* (4th edn) London: Cassell.

Wiley, T. and Merton, B. (2002) *Towards a Contemporary Curriculum*, Leicester: NYA.

Williamson, H. (2005) 'Unstructured work is not youth work', *Young People Now*, 6–12 April 2005. www.cypnow.co.uk/.../Opinion-Unstructured-work-not-youth-work/

Young, K. (2005) *The Art of Youth Work* (2nd edn) Lyme Regis: RHP.

# 7 Evaluation

## Ensuring accountability or improving practice?

*Sue Cooper*

This chapter begins by critically exploring the process of evaluation and the concept of quality in youth work. It will be argued that the dominant discourse fails to address the developmental needs of practitioners or improve practice. Ultimately this fails to improve services, or outcomes for young people. The changing nature of professionalism is considered in the context of the accountability agenda, in particular its effects on professional judgement and professional learning. The chapter then turns to look at what practitioners might do in order to re-engage with the evaluation agenda, exploring the possibilities of an alternative discourse, one that is underpinned by the values of democracy, inclusion and learning. This alternative discourse is much more attuned with youth work principles and practices and therefore one that practitioners are more likely to engage with.

### The process of evaluation

Evaluation is the process used to assess the quality of something, and according to Chelminsky (1997) has three purposes: first, 'accountability', which responds to the demands of funders and stakeholders to meet contractual agreements; second, 'programme development', which focuses on improving the quality of the programme; and third, 'generating knowledge', which aims to develop understanding about what forms of practice are successful. For evaluation to be an effective process in improving outcomes for young people, in developing practitioner's knowledge and skills, and in developing professional knowledge, these three evaluative purposes need equal focus.

It is argued that the process of evaluation within the public services has been corrupted almost entirely by an exclusive focus on accountability, losing its ability to support programme development or generate knowledge and conversely has had a detrimental effect on practice (Issitt and Spence, 2005). The dominance of the accountability model of evaluation has been driven by the neoliberal agenda that prioritizes economy, effectiveness and quality (Rose, 2010), with its emphasis on managerialism. The impact on youth work is evident in the Transforming Youth Work agenda which saw the introduction of externally imposed targets for youth work (DfES, 2002). This shift towards seeing evaluation and indeed quality in terms of quantifiable targets favoured a positivist approach that works on the basis that there are measurable inputs, outputs and outcomes, that there is causality between them, and that a measurement of this will indicate the economy, effectiveness and efficiency of an organization (Ford et al., 2005).

The inappropriateness of this form of evaluation in youth work is striking. Setting measurable outcomes is quite straightforward when the 'product' is tangible, for example, an ASDAN award or a BCU One Star Certificate. However, youth work is a qualitative process; it is concerned with personal and social development and, as such, it is not possible to identify tangible outcomes that lend themselves to measurement. Ord (2007) provides an excellent example of this when he questions what inputs could 'produce' confidence as a youth work outcome. Brent also provides a good example of the intangible nature of youth work outcomes when he describes a young woman's journey in from the periphery as she moved from 'a shadowy appendage of her boy-friend to throw[ing] herself into the life of the Centre' (2004: 70). The pressure to set outcomes which are measurable has led many youth services to focus their attention on those things which lend themselves to being counted, e.g. contacts or accreditations. This presents a very real danger during this period of 're-visioning' youth services and the phrase 'what's measured is what matters' resounds.

The influence of managerialism on the process of evaluation is powerful and the emergence of evidence-based practice and its rapid expansion across a number of areas such as social work, education and youth work needs to be understood against a background of managerialism (Trinder, 2000; Hammersley, 2001). Evidence-based practice has its roots in medicine, and relies upon evidence gathered through scientific experiment, valuing objective knowledge, and devaluing subjective knowledge. Trinder's feminist critique argues that evidence-based practice is 'a covert method of rationing resources, overtly simplistic and constrains professional autonomy' (2000: 3). Davies (2003) supports this view, arguing that evidence-based practice is both a product of managerialism and a means of implementing managerialist agendas. The political obsession with evidence-based practice (Rawnsley, 2001) overlooks the variety of organizational contexts in which practice occurs. It also assumes that there is 'one right way' to practice, further evidencing the dominant positivist approach. Questions concerning what constitutes evidence and who selects it have been raised by many commentators (Smith, 2000; Hammersley, 2001; Davies, 2003) and as Hammersley notes, 'the definition of what is effective, of what counts as "success" will not be something they [professionals] have any control over' (2001).

Despite all of the research that argues against positivism in the social sciences (for example Pring, 2000; Greenwood and Levin, 2005; Whitehead and McNiff, 2006), the reliance on the positivist paradigm in evaluation persists. In fact, some claim we have experienced a 're-emergent scientism, a positivist, evidence-based epistemology' (Denzin and Lincoln, 2005: 8). A good example of this is the Outcome Based Accountability, originally developed by Friedman (2005) in the USA. In the UK it was promoted by the Department of Children, Schools and Families (DCSF) and was taken up by a number of Children's Trusts. In the document *Better Outcomes for Children and Young People: From Talk to Action* (DCSF, 2008), written for directors and lead members of children's services and their key Children's Trust partners, the following statement appears,

> Work is underway to try to understand what works best in 'narrowing the gap' in outcomes, through the Narrowing the Gap Project. This project, funded by DCSF, hosted by the Local Government Association (LGA) and supported by the Improvement and Development Agency (IDeA) is one of a number of initiatives which aims to understand *what action*, if applied *universally and pursued*

*relentlessly*, would make a significant impact on the outcomes of vulnerable groups of children and young people. It is seeking *to identify the simple truths* rooted in evidence across all five outcomes that will assist local authorities and their partners to take effective action to 'narrow the gap' in outcomes between vulnerable children and the rest.

(DCSF, 2008: 6, author's emphasis)

This language leaves the reader in no doubt about the positivist underpinnings of this 'new' approach. McAuley and Cleaver (2006) assert that the four key elements of outcome based accountability are a focus on results, community collaboration, participation by individual citizens, families and children and innovative financial strategies; however, there was little, if any, evidence of how the participatory aspect was implemented or how meaningful it was. What really stands out in McAuley and Cleaver's publication is the emphasis on 'common sense' and a 'simple' approach, particularly in terms of the three common sense performance measures: How much did we do? How well did we do it? And is anyone better off? (Friedman, 2005). The problem is that using terms such as 'common sense' and 'simple' in this way silences any dissenting voices, how can you argue against common sense? Why is it that you do not understand when it is so simple? This is of course a very good example of what was identified in Chapter 2 as 'putting words to work'. The hidden danger of outcome-based accountability is that the collaboration and participation of users is used to legitimize what remains essentially a managerialist process.

## The concept of quality: methodological assumptions

Quality is an elusive concept (Harvey and Green, 1993), with no universally agreed definition (Kelemen, 2003; Watty, 2003) and, interestingly, while '*Many people have commented that they are able to recognise quality when they see it, … [they] find it almost impossible to define*' (Stephenson, 2003, cited in McMillan and Parker, 2005: 153). Different people will have different ways of conceptualizing quality. For example a funder, a senior officer, a practitioner, a service user may all hold different ideas about what quality means. The number and variety of stakeholders involved in youth work brings an increased level of complexity when considering the concept of quality.

Kelemen (2003) offers two opposing perspectives of quality: the managerial perspective and the critical perspective. The managerial perspective views quality as a technical, operational achievement, seeing it as a self-contained entity that can be planned for and controlled with technical and managerial knowledge. This perspective favours a positivist approach in which quality can be studied in a neutral, value-free way through an objective lens. The opposing, critical perspective views quality as a political, cultural and social process. This perspective regards quality as a complex and contested social and political phenomenon, which acquires its meaning via processes of communication in which organizational and societal power play a substantial role. This perspective favours an interpretivist approach which argues quality cannot be studied in a neutral, value-free way through an objective lens. By considering the paradigmatic differences it is possible to shed some light on how these different conceptions of quality impact on what might be considered as appropriate ways of assessing and demonstrating the quality of a particular service, project or piece of work.

*Positivism* is based on the assumptions that scientific knowledge is both accurate and certain (Crotty, 1998) and a belief in the power of scientific knowledge to solve major practical problems (Carr and Kemmis, 1986). The positivist paradigm believes in objective knowledge, that knowledge is value-free, and therefore generalizable and replicable (Wellington, 2000). A positivist methodology seeks to provide explanation and often utilizes quantitative methods. Positivism has its critics; some consider it inappropriate for researching complex issues such as education (Pring, 2000; Whitehead and McNiff, 2006) whilst others cite the lack of recognition and consideration of values as the main problem with the positivist paradigm (Siraj-Blatchford, 1994; O'Donoghue, 2007).

*Interpretivism* emerged as a reaction to positivism. The interpretive paradigm aims to understand the meaning behind something, to explore perspectives and shared meanings and to develop insights into situations (Wellington, 2000). Four main assumptions underpin the interpretive paradigm:

> that knowledge is always situated;
> that people construct their 'lived' reality by attaching specific meanings to their experience;
> that there is always some degree of autonomy; and
> that research involves interaction and negotiation.

(O'Donoghue, 2007)

The ontological position is generally assumed to be relativist, recognizing that there is no one reality, but multiple constructed realities (Denzin and Lincoln, 2005). The epistemological position is subjective and transactional rather than objective. The methodology is generally accepted as naturalistic in approach. Interpretive researchers are interested in the meanings participants attribute to events, in how they make sense of the world, and therefore tend to adopt qualitative methods that capture voice, e.g. interviews, focus groups or diaries, although mixed methods would be compatible. Criticisms of interpretivism generally fall into two categories; first, challenges about validity, reliability and generalizability, which are clearly located in positivist-inspired aspirations (O'Donoghue, 2007). Second, there are those that argue that the value of research that seeks to describe and understand is limited, as it does not in itself bring about change or challenge the status quo (Crotty, 1998; Carr and Kemmis, 1986).

Given the paradigmatic differences between the two opposing conceptions of quality, it is clear to see that the dominant conception is firmly embedded in the positivist paradigm. The adoption of evidenced-based practice and the 'what works?' approach provide examples of this. However, it is argued that the *interpretivist paradigm is a more appropriate choice* than the positivist paradigm for understanding the concept of quality in youth work, for two reasons: the transparency of values; and participation. First, in regard to the transparency of values, positivism claims to be objective and value-free although many would argue that in reality the subjectivity of the researcher is simply hidden or ignored whereas interpretivism accepts that the observer makes a difference to what is observed. The benefit of this openness is that it brings about the need for reflexivity; the interpretivist evaluator must explore the ways in which their involvement influences, acts upon and informs their findings. The interpretivist paradigm allows us to ask questions such as who defines and measures change and for whose benefit this is done (Estrella, 2000). It allows space to raise and challenge hidden agendas (Davies, 2003) and to be open and explicit about the politics, values, and normative aspects of our practice (Abma, 2006). Second, the interpretivist paradigm provides opportunities to raise the voice of participants. In contrast with positivism, which is criticized for silencing voices (Siraj-Blatchford, 1994), the interpretivist paradigm seeks to uncover participants' perspectives. Evaluation underpinned by an interpretivist paradigm enables us to meaningfully engage young people, the community, and importantly, practitioners in the process. This is in contrast to evaluative processes from a positivist paradigm that serves the needs of neoliberalism and moves the locus of power away from the knowledge of practising professionals to the auditors (Davies, 2003). On the contrary, evaluative processes underpinned by an interpretivist paradigm seek to redistribute the power to all those involved.

## The changing nature of evaluation and professionalism

Vedung (2010) argues that recent history of evaluation is best portrayed as a series of waves. In the first wave during the 1960s, she argues, evaluative thinking and practice was driven by a belief that evaluation could make government more rational, scientific and grounded in facts, labelling this as the 'science-driven wave'. Evaluation during this period was carried out by professional academic researchers. Trust and confidence in science to solve social problems began to fade in the 1970s and it was felt that evaluation should be more pluralistic. This led to the second, 'dialogue-oriented wave' – this period called for paradigmatic change, and a constructivist paradigm (Guba and Lincoln, 1989) replaced the positivist paradigm of the science-driven wave. The 1990s saw a growing dissatisfaction with what some people saw as a concept that was 'based too much on biased ideological beliefs, political tactics, pointless bickering, passing fancies and anecdotal knowledge' (Vedung, 2010: 270). The dialogue-oriented wave was replaced by the 'neoliberal wave', characterized by a return to science, with more focus on results and less focus on processes, a fundamental idea in New Public Management. In contrast to the dialogue-oriented wave, the neoliberal wave was customer oriented rather than stakeholder oriented and during this period, evaluation became explicitly linked with accountability, performance measurement and consumer satisfaction. The current wave, according to Vedung (2010), can be seen as the 'evidence wave' and heralds a return to experimentation. Evaluation is concerned with what works, and this can be interpreted as a renaissance, and further embedding, of science and randomized experimentation.

In the context of managerialism, accountability had become a significant management strategy for efficiency and control (Everitt and Hardiker, 1996). Dahlberg et al. argue that:

> Quality and its evaluation can thus become an integral part of a new control system, assuming a policing function, so that 'the power that decentralisation gives away with one hand, evaluation may take back with the other' (Weiler, 1990: 61).
>
> (Dahlberg et al., 2007: 91)

Running alongside, or perhaps underpinning, this use of quality as a technology of control has been the changing nature of professionalism (Ball, 2008) which has radically changed with the advent of neoliberalism. Begun under the Thatcher government, steps were taken to reverse the trend that had led to high professional autonomy during the post-war years, through the introduction of accountability mechanisms. Post-welfarism (Clarke et al., 2000) was accompanied by a shift from a belief that professionalism itself was a reliable guarantor of high quality provision, to a belief that quality was better achieved through externally regulated measures of competency. As a result the professional became viewed more as a technician (Hodkinson and Issitt, 1995). Much of the political discourse of professionalism within the wider social professions seems to place the need for change at the feet of the teacher, the social worker, or the youth worker for their 'failing' practice (Hoyle and John, 1995; Whitty, 2006). This blaming legitimized the centralizing of control and the state's strengthened control of the social professions (Furlong et al., 2000). The trend continued under New Labour, which through a reform and standards agenda took a lead role in shaping the modern professions. However, critics of this conception of 'professional as technician' argue that this oversimplifies the role of the professional. As Young argues in the context of youth work, 'Youth workers do not merely deliver youth work. They define it, interpret it, and develop it' (Young, 1999: 7). The focus on competence is challenged on the basis that 'competence is not and cannot be a fixed concept' (Hodkinson and Issitt, 1995: 148) and that it conceals the place of values.

> Professionals are making complex judgments. These judgments need to be as clear and open as possible – but to pretend that they can be objective and value free is to delude those working in the professions and the users of their services.
>
> (Ibid.)

Everitt and Hardiker (1996) suggest that *practitioners feel alienated from evaluation* as a result of the incompatibility of the positivist approach to the context of their practice. While they make this claim based on case studies drawn from social services, this conflict is also reflected in youth work. The research report *Developing Monitoring and Evaluation in the Third Sector* (Ellis, 2008) confirms that practitioners predominantly believe that evaluation is done mainly for the benefit of funders and regulators, and the assertion is made that externally driven targets and performance indicators reinforce this perception. Others have argued that face-to-face practitioners experience exclusion from the process of evaluation (Issitt and Spence, 2005; Beresford and Branfield, 2006). This separation between practitioners and evaluation is of real concern as it runs the risk of allowing the devaluing of practice knowledge and offers no resistance to the de-professionalization of youth work. Ball uses the term *performativity* to describe the impact of performance management systems on individuals; he argues that 'Performativity invites and incites us to make ourselves more effective, to work on ourselves to improve ourselves and to feel guilty or inadequate if we do not' (2008: 51). This 'improvement' process does little, however, to elevate professional knowledge.

The challenge is to ensure practitioners remain engaged with the process; their absence will offer no opposition to the dominant paradigm. However, in order to do this, practitioners must be able to see a value in evaluation for both themselves and for their practice; this would be achieved if the three evaluative purposes of accountability, professional development and project development (Chelminsky, 1997) were re-balanced. The challenge is to make evaluation useful to practitioners and if we are to do this, then we need to consider an alternative paradigm.

### Reconnecting with evaluation: participatory approaches

A re-balancing of Chelminsky's (1997) threefold purposes of evaluation requires us to adopt approaches to evaluation that equally favour both 'professional' and 'project' development, rather than exclusively focus on accountability. In order to achieve this Dahlberg et al. advocate an interpretivist approach, which emphasizes the importance of '*the discourse of meaning making*':

> Making sense of what is going on within post-modernity is about the construction or making of meaning. We do this, each of us, acting as agents – but always in relation to others, understanding us to be situated in a particular spatial and temporal context.
>
> (2007: 107)

A re-focusing on the evaluative purposes of professional learning and project development (Chelminsky, 1997) enables an entirely different approach to be taken in conceptualizing and undertaking evaluation. The principles of participatory evaluation are in tune with the principles of youth work, as the participatory evaluation process is one that:

> supports and extends participatory models of practice;
> empowers individuals, communities and organizations to analyse and solve their own problems;
> values the knowledge and experience of participants;
> uses learning and education to promote reflection and critical analysis by both project participants and practitioners;
> serves the purpose of improving the programme and the organization in the interests of the users;
> uses participatory methods of obtaining data and generating knowledge, employing a wide range of predominantly qualitative methods, sometimes in combination with quantitative methods; and
> is participatory and collective and that creates better, more in-depth, and more accurate knowledge of the performance and impacts of a practice intervention.
>
> (Jackson and Kassam, 1998)

These principles demonstrate very clearly the huge gulf between the participatory paradigm and the dominant evidence-based, positivist paradigm of evaluation discussed earlier. Estrella (2000) supports these principles as the cornerstones of good practice in evaluation and suggests the all-important feature in the participatory evaluation approach is '*who measures change and who benefits from learning about these changes*'. The purpose, therefore, is not only concerned with tracking change in those directly involved in the change process, but also about ensuring that learning travels up organizational hierarchies and brings about change there as well.

The four main approaches to participatory evaluation are:

#### *Responsive evaluation*

Originally developed by Stake in 1975, responsive evaluation is based on 'what people do naturally to evaluate things: they observe and react' (Stake, 1983: 292). Evaluation is reframed from assessment on the basis of policymakers' goals to an engagement with all stakeholders about the value and meaning of their practice (Abma, 2006). Responsive evaluation takes a naturalistic approach and as such its design needs to be flexible in focus and method. It also assumes value pluralism (Abma and Stake, 2001). Evaluation criteria are derived from the issues of various stakeholders and gradually emerge in conversation with stakeholders rather than being fixed at the outset based on the programme objectives. Responsive evaluation is highly compatible with youth work as the evaluator facilitates the various stakeholders to 'discover ideas, answers, and solutions within their own mind' (Stake and Trumbull, 1982, cited in Luo, 2010: 44), and the evaluation findings generate useful information that can be used to improve the programme.

## Empowerment evaluation

Developed by Fetterman in the 1990s, empowerment evaluation's underlying principles include the extensive participation of project management and staff, funders, community members and other stakeholders in all stages of the evaluation. It seeks to enable collaborative planning and identification of the evidence by which the project will be assessed. Fetterman argues that:

> When evaluators have a vested interest in programs, it enhances their value as critics and evaluators. They will be more constructively critical and supportive of the program because they want the program to work, that is, to succeed.
>
> (2005: 12)

This approach to evaluation aims to empower those that are generally excluded from the decision-making processes of evaluation; they are supported to identify the key issues for evaluations and in shaping the evaluative process, for example, services users become active evaluators rather than passive data providers; the same could be said for practitioners who can also feel excluded from the dominant positivist model of evaluation. The key aim of empowerment evaluation is emancipation, and there is an explicit recognition of the significance of values (Fetterman, 2001). Empowerment evaluation is most appropriate where the program or service being evaluated is aiming to develop self-sufficiency and personal development (Patton, 2008). The alignment with youth work aims and purposes is clear and as a result empowerment evaluation approaches offer youth workers an opportunity to re-engage with meaningful evaluation.

## Practitioner evaluation

Practitioner evaluation was first developed by Stenhouse (1975), who argues that practitioners are the best judges of their practice. Practitioner evaluation sits between empowerment evaluation and reflective practice, and as such is often associated with an action research methodology (Reason and Bradbury, 2000). Practitioner evaluation has three elements:

- the commitment to systematic questioning of one's own practice as a basis for development;
- the commitment and the skills to examine one's own practice; and
- the concern to question and to test theory in practice.

Practitioner evaluation involves practitioners evaluating their own practice or institutions, and by doing so acquiring knowledge that they can use to bring about change in those institutions. There is a growing body of evidence about the effects on practitioners of engaging in research and enquiry in the field of teaching which are transportable to youth work, for example:

> Practitioners gain a better understanding of their practice and ways to improve it (Dadds, 1995).
> Practitioners gain an enhanced sense of the users' perspective of the service (McLaughlin et al., 2004).
> It results in a renewed feeling of pride and excitement about the profession and in a revitalized sense of oneself as a teacher (Dadds, 1995; McLaughlin et al., 2004).
> It restores in practitioners a sense of professionalism and power in the sense of having a voice (McLaughlin et al., 2004).

The difference between this evaluation approach and the dominant positivist approach is striking. Adopting a practitioner evaluation approach could counter the performativity agenda (Ball, 2008) and re-engage practitioners in the process of evaluation as the benefits for them, their practice and ultimately for young people are evident.

### *Appreciative inquiry*

Originally developed by Cooperrider and Srivastava in 1987, appreciative inquiry offers a strength-based collaborative approach to evaluation. This approach involves identifying the things that are done well as opposed to the more traditional starting point of identifying the problem as in action research. Bushe (2007) challenges the view that appreciative inquiry is just action research with a positive question and asserts that it is different as it focuses on generativity rather than problem-solving. Gergen (1994) uses the term 'generativity' to describe the transformative quality of theoretical endeavors. Similarly Schön (1979) introduces the idea of generative metaphors as metaphors that help us gain new perspectives of the world; and Erikson (1950) offers a psychological definition of generativity as the concern with establishing and guiding the next generation. Generativity, in the context of appreciative inquiry, involves the creation of new ideas, perceptions, metaphors or images that are so compelling that they bring about new actions, they shift the way people see the future and they open up new possibilities (Bushe, 2010). Appreciative inquiry is generally accepted to follow a four stage process: discovery, dreaming, design, and delivery (Cooperrider et al., 2008). The process begins with a grounded observation of the 'best of what is', followed by a collective visioning and articulation of 'what might be', ensuring consent to 'what should be' and collectively experimenting with 'what can be'. Over time appreciative inquiry has developed from a focus on evaluation per se, to becoming more aligned with organizational development. As a result Whitney and Trosten-Bloom (2010: 4) argue that appreciative inquiry 'turns command-and-control cultures into communities of discovery and cooperation.'

### The benefits of a participatory approach to evaluation

It is argued that we need to move away from a positivist evaluation paradigm that is linear and closed (Guba and Lincoln, 1989) as this perspective only serves the interests of managerialism (Everitt and Hardiker, 1996). The advantages to using a participatory approach are first that it sets out to acknowledge and elevate the perspectives, voices, and decisions of the least powerful and the most affected stakeholders (Jackson and Kassam, 1998). Second, it promotes a 'doing with' rather than a 'doing to' paradigm. If we are looking to re-engage practitioners in the process of evaluation then using a participatory approach seems highly appropriate. Another key benefit of using a participatory approach is that it recognizes the importance of people's participation in analysing and interpreting change, i.e. learning from experience. Estrella (2000) proposes that participatory evaluation can be used as a self-assessment tool as it enables people to reflect on past experiences, examine current realities, revisit objectives and define future strategies. Using a participatory evaluation approach seems most suited to the aim of ensuring that evaluation not only responds to the need for accountability but also to the need for professional and project development. Keast and Waterhouse (2006) argue that taking a participatory evaluation approach serves to improve change outcomes through providing a mechanism for sustaining change. Patton (2002) asserts that the dual objectives of participatory evaluation are to promote practice improvement and encourage self-evaluation and self-determination. It has been my experience that using a participatory approach can produce opportunities for deep reflection (Cooper, 2010) and Dahlberg et al. (2007) suggest a process that allows practitioners the space to 'make sense of what is going on' through dialogue and critical reflection can increase agency. In other words, the collective spaces that participatory evaluation requires and facilitates offer a place where practitioners can reclaim and re-assert their professional voice and perhaps begin to resist the tightening of professional accountability that is explicitly linked to the prevailing ideology of neoliberalism (Macdonald, 2003).

## Conclusion: so what's to be done?

It has been argued that the dominant discourse of managerialism and positivism are in no small part responsible for the very limited development of participatory approaches; however, adopting a participatory approach to evaluation requires time, effort and energy and in comparison with a positivist model, participatory evaluation is 'positively' hard work. The concern is that practitioners are squashed flat, their reserves depleted. Practitioners in both the statutory and voluntary sectors regularly talk about being over-worked, about the challenges of constant change, and about the ever-increasing demands for data, as well as for evidence of impact.

However, I remain convinced that alternative approaches to evaluation will engage practitioners and through that engagement, practitioners will find both a renewed sense of professional self and replenished energy and enthusiasm for the work. The evidence for this comes from my facilitation of a participatory approach to evaluation in a third sector youth organization (Cooper, 2010). The feedback from the year-long process was that the practitioners highly valued the collective reflection spaces that the approach offered and talked of feeling energized and boosted by the process. I argue it is imperative that managers consider how they might develop opportunities for practitioners to engage in challenging the dominant discourse of evaluation, encouraging developments that support a re-balancing of the evaluative purposes. Some might suggest that this is unrealistic given the managerialist culture and the associated accountability structures, but I am not arguing for an abandonment of the positivist approach – this would be naive given its continued imposition. Rather, I am suggesting that we look to develop parallel participatory approaches that create opportunities for practitioners to engage in collaborative processes that focus on learning and development rather than accountability. By doing this, we can develop alternative paradigms for evaluating practice that encourage a culture that develops practice and practitioners alike, independent of, and additional to, the culture of managerialism. In time perhaps, a counterculture may emerge and begin to challenge it …

## Questions for reflection and discussion

1   In what ways has the accountability agenda impacted on your experience of the evaluation process?
2   How can the participatory methods introduced here be best utilized in your organizations, why would they work well, and what would the benefits be?
3   Which participatory methods would be problematic, what are the barriers, and why would you say these were not working?

## Further reading

Hall, I. and Hall, D. (2004) *Evaluation and Social Research: Introducing Small-scale Practice*, Basingstoke: Palgrave Macmillan.
Rose, J. (2010) 'Monitoring and evaluating youth work', in Jeffs, T. and Smith, M. K. (eds) *Youth Work Practice*. Basingstoke: Palgrave Macmillan, pp. 156–67.
Stake, R. (2004) *Standards-Based and Responsive Evaluation*, London: Sage.
Subhra, G. (2007) 'Reclaiming the evaluation agenda', in Harrison, R., Benjamin, C., Curran, S. and Hunter, R. (eds) *Leading Work with Young People*, London: Sage/Open University Press, pp. 285–98.

## References

Abma, T. (2006) 'The practice and politics of responsive evaluation', *American Journal of Evaluation*, 27(1): 31–43.
Abma, T. and Stake, R. (2001) 'Responsive evaluation, roots and evolution', *New Directions for Evaluation*, vol. 92 (winter): 7–22.
Ball, S. (2008) 'Performativity, privatisation, professionals and the state', in Cunningham, B. (ed.) *Exploring Professionalism*, Bedford Way Papers, London: Institute of Education, pp. 50–72.
Beresford, P. and Branfield, F. (2006) 'Developing inclusive partnerships: user-defined, networking and knowledge – a case study', *Health and Social Care in the Community*, 15(5): 436–44.
Brent, J. (2004) 'Communicating what youth work achieves: the smile and the arch', *Youth and Policy*, Summer, no. 84: 69–73.
Bushe, G. (2010) 'Generativity and the transformational potential of appreciative inquiry', in Zandee, D., Cooperrider, D. L. and Avital, M. (eds) *Organizational Generativity: Advances in Appreciative Inquiry*, Volume 3, Bingley: Emerald. Available at www.gervasebushe.ca/AI_generativity
——(2007) 'Appreciative inquiry is not (just) about the positive', *OD Practitioner*, 39(4): 30–35.
Carr, W. and Kemmis, S. (1986) *Becoming Critical: Education, Knowledge and Action Research*, London: Falmer Press.
Chelminsky, E. (1997) 'Thoughts for a new evaluation society', *Evaluation*, 3(1): 97–118.
Clarke, J., Gewirtz, S. and McClaughlin, E. (eds) (2000) *New Managerialism, New Welfare*, London: Sage/Open University Press.
Cooper, S. (2010) 'Reconnecting with evaluation: some encouraging signs coming from the implementation of a participatory approach', Paper delivered to the TAG conference at Durham University, July.

Cooperrider, D. and Srivastava, S. (1987) 'Appreciative inquiry in organizational life', in Woodman, R. and Pasmore, W. (eds) *Research in Organizational Change and Development, vol. 1*, Greenwich, CT: JAI Press, pp. 129–69.

Cooperrider, D., Whitney, D. and Stavros, J. (2008) *Appreciative Inquiry Handbook* (2nd edn) Brunswick, OH: Crown Custom Publishing.

Crotty, M. (1998) *The Foundations of Social Research: Meaning and Perspective in the Research Process*, London: Sage.

Dadds, M. (1995) *Passionate Enquiry and School Development: Story About Teacher Action Research*, London: Routledge.

Dahlberg, G., Moss, P. and Pence, A. (2007) *Beyond Quality in Early Childhood Education and Care* (2nd edn) London: Routledge.

Davies, B. (2003) 'Death to critique and dissent? The policies and practices of new managerialism and of "evidence-based practice"', *Gender and Education*, 15(1): 91–103.

DCSF (2008) *Better Outcomes for Children and Young People: From Talk to Action*, London: DCSF.

Denzin, N. and Lincoln, Y. (2005) (eds) *The Sage Handbook of Qualitative Research* (3rd edn) London: Sage.

DfES (2002) *Transforming Youth Work: Resourcing Excellent Youth Services*, London: HMSO.

Ellis, J. (2008) *Accountability and Learning: Developing Monitoring and Evaluation in the Third Sector: Research briefing*, London: Charities Evaluation Services.

Erikson, E. H. (1950) *Childhood and Society*, New York: Norton.

Estrella, M. (2000) 'Learning from change', in Estrella, M., Blauert, J., Campilan, D., Gaventa, J., Gonsalves, J., Guijt, I., Johnson, D. and Ricafort, R. (eds) *Learning From Change: Issues and Experiences in Participatory Monitoring and Evaluation*, London: Intermediate Technology Publications, pp. 1–14.

Everitt, A. and Hardiker, P. (1996) *Evaluating for Good Practice*, Basingstoke: Macmillan Press.

Fetterman, D. (2005) 'A window into the heart and soul of empowerment evaluation: looking through the lens of empowerment evaluation principles', in Fetterman, D. and Wandersman, A. (eds) *Empowerment Evaluation Principles in Practice*, New York: Guilford Press, pp. 1–26.

——(2001) 'The transformation of evaluation into collaboration: A vision of evaluation in the 21st century', *American Journal of Evaluation*, 22(3): 381–85.

Ford, K., Hunter, R., Merton, B. and Waller, D. (2005) *Leading and Managing Youth Work*, Leicester: NYA.

Friedman, M. (2005) *Trying Hard is Not Good Enough: How to Produce Measurable Improvements for Customers and Communities*, Oxford: Trafford Publications.

Furlong, J., Barton, L., Miles, S., Whiting, C. and Whitty, G. (2000) *Teacher Education in Transition: Reforming Professionalism?* Buckingham: Open University Press.

Gergen, K. (1978) 'Toward generative theory', *Journal of Personality and Social Psychology*, vol. 36: 1344–60.

——(1994) *Realities and Relationships: Soundings in Social Construction*, Cambridge, MA: Harvard University Press.

Greenwood, D. and Levin, M. (2005) 'Reform of the social services, and of universities through action research', in Denzin, N. and Lincoln, Y. (eds) *The Sage Handbook of Qualitative Research* (3rd edn) London: Sage, pp. 43–64.

Guba, E. and Lincoln, Y. (1989) *Fourth Generation Evaluation*, London: Sage.

Hammersley, M. (2001) 'Some questions about evidence-based practice in education', Paper presented at the symposium on 'Evidence-based Practice in Education' at the Annual Conference of the British Educational Research Association, University of Leeds, 13–15 September.

Harvey, L. and Green, D. (1993) 'Defining quality', *Assessment and Evaluation in Higher Education*, 18(1): 9–34.

Hodkinson, P. and Issitt, M. (eds) (1995) *The Challenge of Competence: Professionalism through Vocational Education and Training*, London: Cassell.

Hoyle, E. and John, P. (1995) *Professional Knowledge and Professional Practice*, London: Cassell.

Issitt, M. and Spence, J. (2005) 'Practitioner knowledge and evidence-based research, policy and practice', in *Youth and Policy*, Summer, no. 88: 63–82.

Jackson, E. and Kassam, Y. (eds) (1998) *Knowledge Shared: Participatory Evaluation in Development Cooperation*, London: IDRC/Kumarian Press.

Keast, R. and Waterhouse, J. (2006) 'Participatory evaluation: a missing component in the sustainable social change equation for public services', *Strategic Change*, vol. 15: 23–35.

Kelemen, M. (2003) *Managing Quality: Managerial and critical perspectives*, London: Sage.

Luo, H. (2010) 'The role for an evaluator: a fundamental issue for evaluation of education and social programs', *International Education Studies*, 3(2): 42–50.

Macdonald, C. (2003) 'Forward via the past? Evidence-based practice as strategy in social work', *The Drawing Board: An Australia Review of Public Affairs*, 3(3): 123–42.

McAuley, C. and Cleaver, D. (2006) *Improving Service Delivery Through Outcome-Based Accountability*, London: Improvement and Development Agency for Local Government.

McLaughlin, C., Black-Hawkins, K. and McIntyre, D. (2004) *Researching Teachers, Researching Schools, Researching Networks: A Summary of the Literature*. Accessed at networkedlearning.ncsl.org.uk/.../commissioned-research-cambs-final-total-edited-su-979db.doc

McMillan, W. and Parker, M. (2005) 'Quality is bound up with our values: evaluating the quality of mentoring programmes', *Quality in Higher Education*, 11(2): 151–60.

Morris, E. (2001) *Professionalism and Trust: The Future of Teachers and Teaching*, London: DfES/Social Market Foundation.

O'Donoghue, T. (2007) *Planning Your Qualitative Research Project: An Introduction to Interpretivist Research in Education*, Abingdon: Routledge.

Ord, J. (2007) *Youth Work Process, Product and Practice: Creating an Authentic Curriculum in Work with Young People*, Lyme Regis: RHP.

Patton, M. (2008) *Utilization-focussed Evaluation* (4th edn) London: Sage.

——(2002) *Qualitative Research and Evaluation Methods* (3rd edn) London: Sage.

Pring, R. (2000) *Philosophy of Educational Research*, London: Continuum.

Rawnsley, A. (2001) *Servant of the People: The Inside Story of New Labour*, Harmondsworth: Penguin.

Reason, P. and Bradbury, H. (2000) *Handbook of Action Research: Participatory Inquiry and Practice*, London: Sage.

Rose, J. (2010) 'Monitoring and evaluating youth work', in Jeffs, T. and Smith, M. K. (eds) *Youth Work Practice*, Basingstoke: Palgrave Macmillan, pp. 156–67.

Schön, D. A. (1979) 'Generative metaphor: a perspective on problem-setting in social policy', in Ortony, A. (ed.) *Metaphor and Thought*, Cambridge: Cambridge University Press, pp. 354–83.

Siraj-Blatchford, I. (1994) *Praxis Makes Perfect: Critical Educational Research for Social Justice*, Derbyshire: Education Now Books

Smith, D. (2000) 'The limits of positivism revisited', Paper delivered at the 'What Works as Evidence for Practice? The Methodological Repertoire in an Applied Discipline' seminar, Cardiff, 27 April. ESRC funded.

Stake, R. (1975) 'To evaluate an arts program', in Robert E. Stake (ed.) *Evaluating the Arts in Education: A Responsive Approach*, Columbus, OH: Charles E. Merrill, pp. 13–38.

——(1983) 'Program evaluation, particularly responsive evaluation,' in G. Madaus, M. Scriven and D. Stufflebeam (eds) *Evaluation Models: Viewpoints on Educational and Human Services Evaluation*, Boston, MA: Kluwer-Nijhoff, pp. 287–310.

Stenhouse, L. (1975) *An Introduction to Curriculum Development and Research*, London: Heinemann.

Trinder, L. (ed.) (2000) *Evidence-based Practice: A Critical Appraisal*, Oxford: Blackwell Science.

Vedung, E. (2010) 'Four waves of evaluation', *Evaluation*, 16(3): 263–77.

Watty, K. (2003) 'When will academics learn about quality?' *Quality in Higher Education*, 9(3): 213–21.

Wellington, J. (2000) *Educational Research: Cotemporary Issues and Practical Approaches*, London: Continuum Books.

Whitehead, J. and McNiff, J. (2006) *Action Research: Living Theory*, London: Sage.

Whitney, D. and Trosten-Bloom, A. (2010) *The Power of Appreciative Inquiry. A Practical Guide to Positive Change* (2nd edn) San Francisco: Berrett-Koehler.

Whitty, G. (2006) 'Teacher professionalism in a new era', Paper presented at the first General Teaching Council for Northern Ireland Annual Lecture, Belfast, March.

Young, K. (1999) *The Art of Youth Work*, Lyme Regis: Russell House.

# 8  Re-balancing supervision

*Sue Cooper, with Pauline Grace, Graham Griffiths and Kate Sapin*

This chapter sets out to identify how the process of supervision has fundamentally changed as a result of the neoliberal policy context and managerialism. It will argue that the technical-rational approach to managerial supervision has resulted in it becoming a process of surveillance rather than a process of reflective practice. We present a social constructivist approach (Parton, 2003; Hair and O'Donoghue, 2009) as an alternative paradigm that can enable supervisors and supervisees to claim back the space to reflectively review their work, and where the three functions of supervision can be balanced. We conclude by considering alternative modes of supervision: peer, group, and team, to offer the reader some creative ways of addressing the conflicting demands placed upon supervision.

## The complexity of supervision

Supervision is a generic term that 'continues to be subject to many different interpretations by practitioners and managers' (Beddoe, 2010: 1283). It includes a number of related tasks and relationships, which include: 'managerial supervision', the supervision of staff by the manager; 'non-managerial supervision', the supervision of staff by someone other than their manager, often external to the organization; and 'peer supervision', supervision with and by colleagues. Managerial supervision takes place in a 1–1 relationship whereas the other modes can occur in 1–1 or in group settings. Supervision is a process and the process is context specific involving personal, professional and organizational issues, all of which will impact on the style and approach to supervision. In this chapter, we begin by focusing on managerial supervision, and in particular how managerialism has impacted upon the process of managerial supervision, and conclude by suggesting that other types of supervision can assist in a rebalancing of the primary functions of supervision. It is important to understand the complexity of the process of supervision, as the deeper our understanding of the issues involved the more likely we are to be able to construct and enact a process that effectively supports good practice. A level of complexity arises because of the relational dimension of supervision: 'Above all it [supervision] involves attitudes and feelings of a supervisor in a relationship with another person' (Marchant, 1987: 40). An effective supervisory relationship relies on the foundations of trust, openness and mutuality (Hawkins and Shohet, 2006), the very things that have been undermined by managerialism.

At its most fundamental, Tegg (1990) claimed supervision contains the twin purposes of, first, establishing the accountability of the worker to the organization, and second, to promote the worker's development as a professional person, what Marken and

Payne (1987) referred to as 'ensuring' and 'enabling'. A definition of supervision which encompasses these two functions is offered by Brown and Bourne, who consider managerial supervision as the primary means by which 'an agency-designated supervisor enables staff, individually and collectively; and ensures standards of practice' (1996: 9).

Developing this, Kadushin (1992) suggests that there are three purposes of supervision: 'administrative', 'educational' and 'supportive'. However, his work was arguably based on the traditional expert–apprenticeship model, which placed the supervisor in a superior role as the transmitter of knowledge. Kadushin therefore did not place sufficient emphasis on the two-way process of supervision, recognize 'the facilitation of learning', or give enough credit to the supervisee's prior knowledge. As Brown and Bourne (1996) argued, the supervisee is an active participant in the intentional process of supervision. Inskipp and Proctor (1993) identified three similar purposes; the first was the formative purpose that focussed on the development of the worker. The second was the normative purpose: this attended to the ongoing monitoring and evaluation and assessment of practice. Third was the restorative purpose, ensuring the worker is adequately refreshed and re-creative. A premise of this chapter is that supervision has three essential functions, namely 'restorative/supportive', 'formative/educative' and 'normative/managerial'; and that the process itself must be 'two-way'.

It is also argued that all three components need to be incorporated and addressed within supervision if it is to be effective. As Smith (2005) suggests, it is not only helpful to think of the three elements as interlinked, but to recognize that removing any one element from the process would result in supervision becoming potentially less satisfying to both parties and less effective overall.

Acknowledging the contrasting functions, Ingram and Harris (2001) suggest that effective line management supervision needs to find a balance between the competing demands of the organizational needs and the worker's needs, as well as taking account of the relationship between the worker and manager. They rightly point out that tensions can arise between the demands of the young-person-centred nature of the profession, set against an organization's need for accountability, and for the organization to fulfil its managerial function. A further tension is introduced with an appreciation of the individual supervisee's specific circumstances, strengths and professional development requirements.

The earliest exploration of supervision in youth work was by Tash (1967), and she was largely responsible for establishing the centrality of developmental supervision to youth work practice. She saw 'The supervisory function (while sometimes helping them [supervisees] in relation to their employers) was not to see that they did their work properly, but to help them understand their work at the points at which the workers indicated that they needed help' (Tash, 1967: 16). She was, however, not referring to managerial supervision, as one of the assumptions underpinning her developmental approach was that the supervisor had no authority over the supervisee. We would not argue supervision can, or even should be completely removed from its 'normative' or 'ensuring' function. But Tash does 'hold up a mirror' to contemporary supervisors in youth work, and we will shortly argue the pendulum has swung considerably away from a developmental focus towards a managerial focus in contemporary supervision.

As Bradley and Höjer (2009) found in their comparative study of social work supervision in England and Sweden, whilst all three functions of supervision were addressed, in England, the emphasis has been for some time on accountability. Similarly, Ash recognizes the risk of this unbalanced agenda, reminding us of the important link between good supervision and effective practice, and highlighting that it is only 'reflective supervision [which] produces reflective practice' (1995: 26).

## Changing times: the impact of managerialism

As has been previously discussed in earlier chapters (in particular Chapter 2), the neo-liberal agenda and the resulting managerialism has significantly impacted on the management of youth work. In part this is characterized by a shift of power from practising professionals to auditors and policy-makers (Davies, 2003). Increasingly public sector organizations were seen as inefficient and professions as incapable of regulating their own practice. The solution to these apparent problems was seen as the adoption of managerialism, including a system of prescribed outcomes, micro-management and external audit (Power, 1997). It was the development of an audit culture that significantly impacted on the process of supervision within the social professions. An audit culture necessitates a focus on outcomes and requires a system to monitor those outcomes. In this situation where there is a preoccupation with oversight of practice, supervision becomes 'a monitoring mechanism for administrative accountability' (Tsui, 1997: 197). Managerialism has brought about conditions where workers find themselves practising in pressured environments in which they are then pressured to meet targets (Seden and McCormick, 2011). Payne and Scott argued that whilst acknowledging accountability was an important 'part' of supervision, supervision was not 'merely a vehicle for accountability to the organization' (1982: 8). In contemporary practice however, supervision appears to be almost exclusively concerned with such accountability (Beddoe, 2010).

There is resurgence of interest in the concept of supervision in the social professions (Bradley and Höjer, 2009; Beddoe, 2010) which has even been identified in the prominent and influential Laming report, commenting on both the importance of, as well as the weaknesses in, the practice of supervision:

> Supervision is the cornerstone of good social work practice and should be seen to operate effectively at all levels of the organization. In Haringey, the provision of supervision may have looked good on paper, but in practice it was woefully inadequate for many of the front-line staff. This must change. The same is true for the police and the health services.
>
> (Laming, 2003: para. 1.59)

However this renewed emphasis is open to interpretation. Does it indicate that the way in which the supervisory process enabled and supported workers to deliver in the messy and complex contexts of practice (Schön, 1987) was woefully inadequate or was it suggesting that there had been insufficient monitoring of practice? It is doubtful that what was being emphasized is a commitment to 'balanced and reflective' supervision. Bradley and Höjer argue that whilst the importance of supervision has gained ground within the statutory services, it is in a more administrative, management-dominated format (2009: 74). The Children's Workforce Development Council (CWDC) continued this revitalization when they stated: 'High quality supervision is one of the most important drivers in ensuring positive outcomes for people who use social care and children's services' in their publication 'Providing Effective Supervision' (CWDC, 2007: 2). Whilst some might see this statement as a positive step towards reasserting the importance of effective supervision as a place to develop the practice and the practitioner, we argue that this revitalization of, and re-emphasis on, supervision is more concerned with accountability, which promotes increased surveillance of professional practice (Beddoe 2010). Perhaps it was as Johns (2001) suggested, that 'supervision is at risk of becoming another technology of surveillance and becomes an opportunity to shape the practitioner into organizationally preferred ways of practice, even whilst veiled as being in the practitioner's best interests' (ibid.: 140).

It is unlikely that this interpretation of supervision is going to be experienced positively by both supervisors and supervisees, and as a result commitment to the process will be or indeed has been reduced. This situation in social work is paradoxically described by Sawdon and Sawdon as resulting in a situation whereby 'supervision is both central and marginal to the practice of social work' (1995: 3). They argue that supervision is central because the most important resource for the organization is the personal resources of the staff. However, it is marginal because the practice and purpose of supervision was confused, misunderstood and undervalued; and they go on to suggest that some of this apathy towards supervision was as a result of the unbalanced focus on the three functions, with the accountability function becoming dominant. Here lies the problem, for, at a time of continual change and uncertainty, criticality and reflexivity are core components of effective practice and yet supervision that privileges accountability over learning and support is unlikely to promote development in these areas. For this reason, it is in important to look again at our supervisory practice and make every effort to rebalance the three functions of supervision.

## Overcoming the barriers: reconstructing supervision

In this section we will look in more detail at some of the reasons why the functions of supervision can become unbalanced, focussing on the issues of trust, the narrow interpretation of accountability – solely in terms of accountability to the organization – and the importance of a social constructivist perspective instead of the dominant technical-rational approach to service delivery.

### *The issue of trust*

The issue of trust is an important factor in shaping any relationship, and the supervisory relationship is no different. As alluded to earlier in Chapter 4, managerialism, and in particular its associated audit culture, has eroded trust at a number of levels: between government and managers, between managers and practitioners and between practitioners and services users (Power, 1997; O'Neill, 2002; Davies, 2003; Evetts, 2006). Trust is an attitude that accepts risk, and involves vulnerability (Smith, 2001). This would appear to be in opposition to the technical-rational approach to practice that is risk-averse, prioritizes control and leaves little room for the practitioner to express doubt. Trust, however, cannot be demanded or enforced; it depends on voluntary reciprocity. It is helpful for managers to heed the advice of Proctor:

> It is most useful to start with the assumptions that workers in the human service professions can be relied on to want to monitor their own practice,[1] to learn to develop competence and to respond to support and encouragement.
>
> (Proctor, 1988; in Hawkins and Shohet, 2006: 49)

Austin and Hopkins (2004) claim that although the main responsibility for establishing trust in the supervisory relationship lies with the supervisor, the context of the supervision cannot be ignored. The dominant performativity culture will therefore impact on the supervisory relationship. Hawkins and Shohet (2006) use the term 'hidden client' to represent the influence organizational culture can have on the supervisory relationship. They suggest that just raising the issue of culture within the relationship can potentially lead to some degree of change. Moving away from the risk averse culture of managerialism would allow the supervisory process to become a space where there is a willingness to take risks and to learn from mistakes. This shift would require the development of high levels of trust. However, in turn this would enable the enhancement of the social and intellectual capital of the institution and its members (Hargreaves, 1999a and 2001, cited in Avis, 2005: 213). This is a very different ethos to that of the 'blame culture' found within managerialism and change, if achievable, will not be swift or straightforward. Building trust is an evolutionary process that is directly related to how issues of power are dealt with. But Austin and Hopkins suggest that 'if supervisors hold themselves, as well as their supervisees, accountable in the relationship, trust in the relationship will increase' (2004: 30). Taking this perspective enables both supervisees and supervisors to become active agents of change.

### Narrow confines of accountability

Raising an awareness of the narrow construction of accountability, within managerialist supervision, aids the process of reconstructing alternative ways of conceptualizing supervision. Accountability which reduces risk-taking consequently hinders the development of creative problem solving (Avis, 2005). Accountability is narrowly defined as being 'accountable to the organization' and to the confines of pre-specified outcomes and targets. Accountability viewed in this way can be seen to reduce or even replace autonomy (Evans, 2008) and results in performance becoming 'conformance' to a 'standardization of practice' (Evetts, 2005). This approach to accountability shifts the focus from what practitioners can do in delivering services to what they cannot do (Chaharbaghi, 2010).

However, if we challenge this narrow construction of accountability, from being about the meeting of prescribed targets, to a more holistic construction in which accountability can be defined as:

> the process of taking responsibility for your own behaviour and its impact on yourself and others. First, it is a commitment to tell a true story about your work ... Second, it is a commitment to take responsible actions.
>
> (Austin and Hopkins 2004: 24–25)

Then we can also challenge the conception of managerial supervision as being about checking performance. This begins to lead to a re-balancing of the three functions of supervision; administration, education and support. A power shift is required, however, if accountability is to be viewed more holistically, a shift which expands the parameters of accountability within supervision beyond 'being accountable to the organization', to being accountable to the client, and to one's self, as well as to the wider profession.

As a result of this shift the supervisee becomes a more active participant in the supervision and the role of the supervisor changes from 'overseer' to 'problem-poser'.

A focus on delivery according to prescribed targets and pre-specified plans is likely to negatively impact on open dialogue, whereas a focus on problem-posing requires it. As Sapin argues, supervision in youth work should be congruent with the practice of youth work; in others words, it should be 'based on dialogue and problem-posing' (2009: 187). Drawing on Freire (1972), she argues for a process in which both supervisor and supervisee are open to learning through dialogue, where both are responsible for the process. Kadushin and Harkness in their discussion of social work supervision also argue for 'both model and method' which are Socratic in essence and founded upon the interpersonal dialogic relationship (2002: 152). Kögler also suggests that it is only 'the liberating, problematising, innovative, and unpredictable potential of conversation, which is capable of leading us to new insights and critical self-reflection through experiencing the other' (1999: 1).

However, alongside this Kögler reminds us that power can be a constraint on open conversation and has the potential to undermine the critical capacity of dialogue. It is therefore essential for supervisors and supervisees to raise the issue of power, as Brown and Bourne argue: 'Issues to do with power, and how it is managed, lie at the heart of supervision and the supervisory relationship' (1996: 32). Power exists on a number of levels: personal, cultural and structural (Thompson, 1997), and needs to be addressed at each of these levels. If we fail to take account of the context in which the supervisory relationship sits, in other words, if we fail to comprehend the impact of power at the institutional and policy levels, 'the system dynamics', we are at risk of becoming stuck in 'cycles of blaming and self-defence: the enemy is always out there, and problems are always caused by someone else' (Bolman and Deal, 1997: 27). The focus of conversations within supervision should be open to consideration of the external organizational context, particularly the impact of the contemporary political and economic circumstances. Supervision can provide an opportunity to explore these issues as a means of developing ways to understand the conflicting demands of different parts of the organization and community, particularly the young people.

Senge (1994) argues that when dialogue is joined with systems thinking, there is the possibility of creating a language more suited to dealing with complexity, and focusing on structural issues and power. Essentially, the systemic thinking method (Senge, 1994: 81) can be seen as the recognition that every decision and action will inevitably have an impact upon something or someone else within the organization. An organization committed to learning, being open, and operating in a climate of mutual respect and trust will acknowledge the influence and invisible presence of parties other than the supervisor–supervisee within the supervisory relationship (Hawkins and Shohet, 2006).

### Social constructivist approach to supervision

Finally, in this section, we offer a critique of the dominant technical-rational approach to managerial supervision and suggest that a social constructivist approach should be developed as an alternative paradigm. The technical-rational discourse associated with managerialism is underpinned by the positivist (or post-positivist) paradigm. It assumes that there is 'one truth', one way of practising, that we can discover this through experimentation and we can then generalize 'best practice' elsewhere. It values objectivity over subjectivity and standardization over creativity (Parton and O'Byrne, 2000). Although the appropriateness of a positivist paradigm for practice has been contested (Everitt and Hardiker 1996; Dahlberg et al., 2007) it continues to influence supervision literature and practice (Kadushin and Harkness, 2002). However, Schön (1987) argued that such a positivist model of practice fails to capture how practitioners operate and how they 'know' in practice. The everyday problems they are faced with are not presented in a way which easily fit technical-rational approaches. Real world problems do not come well-formed but, on the contrary, present themselves as messy and indeterminate.

Moving from a positivist paradigm to a social constructivist paradigm provides an opportunity to emphasize process, the plurality of both knowledge and voice, and the relational quality of knowledge (Parton, 2003). Knowing is a social and dialogical process; viewing supervision through a social constructivist lens places central importance on the concept of reflexivity (Taylor and White, 2000) and requires us to '*continual[ly] attempt to place one's premises into question and to listen to alternative framings of reality in order to grapple with the potentially different outcomes arising out of different points of view*' (Parton, 2003: 9). It highlights the importance of entering into dialogue and allows us to view supervision as a collaborative process, rather than a hierarchical one. It opens the space to allow the questioning of the structural and policy influences, and impacts, on practice and seeks a position of 'informed not-knowing' (Laird, 1998: 23), rather than expert knowledge, encouraging a two-way learning dialogue. Using a social constructivist lens enables supervisors to shape a supervisory relationship that encourages transparency, collaboration, and an exchange of ideas (Hair and O'Donoghue, 2009). Supervisors, therefore, are encouraged to be tentative about their own knowledge, and curious about the knowledge of the supervisee. When this happens, conversations between supervisors and supervisees can be critically reflective 'dialogic-reflexive interactions' (Walker, 2001: 36).

Within the constraints of the current climate, we argue that it 'is possible' to work 'towards' a re-balancing of the functions of supervision; particularly if trust is developed, the confines of accountability are widened and a social constructivist perspective is adhered to. There are also some helpful *models*; for example, Hawkins and Shohet's (2006) seven-eyed process model which identifies seven modes of supervision: focus on the client, focus on the supervisee's interventions, focus on the supervisee–client relationship, focus on supervisee, focus on supervisory relationship, focus on supervisor's self-reflection, and focus on the wider practice context. And there is Ingram and Harris's (2001) three-circle model: the needs of the organization, the developmental needs of staff and the developmental needs of the young people. These models can assist us in thinking about the degree of balance in the supervision we give or receive. We can also consider alternative or additional modes of supervision that have the potential to offer practitioners the restorative and formative space needed to sustain practice and practitioners during ever-changing, ever more complex times.

## Alternative modes of supervision

In this final section we explore peer, group and team supervision as alternative or additional modes of supervision. The advantages and disadvantages of these modes will be examined in terms of their potential to support practitioners during times of uncertainty and change. Adopting any one of these complementary models of supervision offers the supervisor and supervisee an opportunity to address the managerial shift in supervision.

## Peer supervision

Peer supervision is defined as supervision among and led by peers (Bond and Holland, 1998; Hawkins and Shohet, 2006). It can take place in one-to-one settings, triad settings or group settings. The principles of peer supervision are seen as the collegial relationship, the focus of accountability being towards the profession, and its orientation towards professional development and support. Zorga et al. (2001) highlight the 'potential for learning' as a key benefit of peer supervision. There is also considerable potential for the 'support' function, including the sustaining of one's professional identity in this mode of supervision. This may become increasingly important in light of the moves towards interprofessional working contexts, where one's line manager may not be from a youth work background.

Peer supervision, however, does have its own challenges, and does require individuals to have a level of knowledge and understanding about the nature of supervision (Wilkerton, 2006). There are a number of difficulties associated with one-to-one peer supervision; these include the competing need of supervisees for supervision, and the difficulties peers may have in challenging each other in terms of promoting development, competition or common praising (Hawkins and Shohet, 2006). As a result there is a danger of slipping into consensus collusion (Butterworth 1998). Clough (1995: 105–6) suggests that these difficulties may be overcome by ensuring 'clarity as to the nature of the relationship, and the responsibility for determining the agenda and action'.

## Group supervision

Supervision can be provided in a group setting, and Proctor's (2008) typology provides a good starting point to understand the different types of group supervision. Proctor identifies four types:

1   *authoritative group supervision* where the supervisor supervises each supervisee in turn and manages the group;
2   *participative group supervision* where the supervisor is responsible for supervising but also for facilitating the development of supervisees as co-supervisors;
3   *co-operative group supervision* where the role of the supervisor is group facilitator, and supervisees contract to co-supervise; and
4   *peer group supervision* in which the members take shared responsibility to supervise and be supervised as described above.

(Proctor, 2008: 32)

Of these four types, we argue that within a youth work context, the participative or co-operative group supervision would be most suited to provide supervision alongside managerial supervision, as this mode requires a joint commitment from both supervisees and supervisors to share power and responsibility. Although as Proctor herself recognizes, the types are not clearly distinct from each other and it is likely that groups will move between types at different times. Group supervision provides an opportunity for each member to learn from others through sharing knowledge, hearing different perspectives, and discussing issues, both common and unique to each of them (Bogo et al., 2004). Kadushin and Harkness (2002) also claim that group supervision, particularly peer group supervision, offers the worker a greater measure of autonomy.

Group supervision provides a collective space at a time when 'the policy technologies of market, management and performativity leave no space for an autonomous or collective ethical self' (Ball, 2003: 226). The potential empowering nature of groups can offer a challenge to the dominant culture of performativity; if problems are experienced in relation to others' struggles, practitioners may understand them more as part of professional development than as an indicator of personal inadequacy (Kadushin, 1992). In other words, group supervision may be able to support practitioners to '*redefine individuals' problems as shared political experiences*' (Preston-Shoot, 2007). As Doel and Sawdon suggest:

> The philosophy of groupwork is based on a belief in the power of the collective solution ... It is a place where individuals can find their voices, individually or together, learn together and challenge together.
>
> (1999: 25)

Other benefits of group supervision are that it makes more economic use of supervisor time and expertise (Hawkins and Shohet, 2006) and reduces the risk of developing dependency on the supervisor (Bogo et al., 2004). However, group supervision brings some significant challenges, particularly for the supervisor, as another layer of complexity is added to relationships, roles, and expectations (Kuechler, 2006). Groups can be uncomfortable places for some people; the group is a semi-public space and this visibility can be challenging and 'the sense of belonging ... can just as easily degenerate into feelings of not belonging' (Doel and Sawdon, 1999: 15). It is vital to develop and maintain a productive group climate and process where practitioners view themselves as interdependent and interactive in the shared pursuit of learning (Kadushin and Harkness, 2002).

Challenges to this productive climate are generally seen in terms of group dynamics, which range from competition and rivalry, to group collusion in terms of 'groupthink' (Janis, 1972) (characterized as a deterioration of, mental efficiency, reality testing, and moral judgment, that results from in-group pressures). Threats to productive group conditions must be identified and resolved in order for group supervision to be useful (Bogo et al., 2004). Despite some of these challenges, we would argue that, as group supervision is congruent with youth work practice, and therefore youth workers are often skilled group workers, they are well placed to make effective use of this mode of supervision.

## Team supervision

The final mode of supervision we will explore is team supervision. This is group supervision but within a team, and it is usually the team leader who holds the supervisor role. It is likely that team supervision would align with Proctor's authoritative or participative group supervision type, although the power of the team leader does need to be acknowledged. This mode of supervision can support collaboration (Hyrkas and Appelqvist-Schmidlechner, 2003) but it can also reflect the current tensions and unresolved dynamics of the team (Proctor, 2008). Team supervision can offer a constructive arena for critical dialogue regarding current policy implementation, as well as enable the team members to actively participate in visioning the future on the ground. In uncertain times it can support communication and reduce anxiety but, as with group supervision more generally, the supervisor will need to skilfully develop and maintain a productive group climate and process to enable this to happen. Using an appreciative inquiry approach, which is a strength-based collaborative approach, within team supervision, can enable people to feel energized and this can raise morale (see Chapter 7 for more details about appreciative enquiry and its use in evaluation).

Team supervision could also be beneficial when the team is composed of different professionals, as it can lead to a greater understanding of the different professional perspectives, values and culture. It is, however, important that the supervisor makes clear that it is plurality that is sought, not consensus. Team supervision in the context of interprofessionalism can support collaboration and communication, as confirmed by Hyrkas and Appelqvist-Schmidlechner (2003). They found that team supervision was able to shift the focus of supervision from individual clients to team strategies, processes and performance and in doing so was able to resolve communication issues at the deeper level.

*To conclude*, it is evident that neoliberalism has had a negative impact on the 'formative and educative' and 'restorative and supportive' functions of supervision. This results from the narrow construction of accountability, the imposition of an audit culture and performativity, as well as the technical-rational approach to delivering services. In the present climate of savage cuts to the funding of youth services, we argue that the need for effective supervision is even more essential to sustain practice and practitioners. We argue that adopting a social constructivist approach to supervision and to the concept of accountability enables us to construct a more balanced supervision process. We suggest that by offering some alternative approaches that may be used in tandem with managerial supervision, it may be possible to support, empower and sustain practitioners through the uncertain and tumultuous times ahead.

## Questions for reflection and discussion

1   Can you identify from your experience of being supervised and/or being a supervisor how the process of supervision has been dominated by the accountability agenda?
2   Can you think of ways in which you can rebalance your supervision process (either as a supervisee or supervisor) to better enable the development and supportive functions to be fulfilled?
3   How can the alternative modes of supervision be utilized within your organization to further support and develop practice?

## Note

1 See Chapter 3 for an exploration of humanist management theory which emphasizes the importance of practitioners' motivation.

## Further reading

Austin, M. and Hopkins, K. (eds) (2004) *Supervision as Collaboration in the Human Services: Building a Learning Culture*, London: Sage.
Davys, A. and Beddoe, L. (2010) *Best Practice in Professional Supervision: A Guide for the Helping Professions*, London: Jessica Kingsley.
Hawkins, P. and Shohet, R. (2006) *Supervision in the Helping Professions* (3rd edn) Berkshire: Open University Press.

## References

Ash, E. (1995) 'Supervision: taking account of feelings', in Pritchard, J. (ed.) *Good Practice in Supervision*, London: Jessica Kingsley, pp. 20–30.

Austin, M. and Hopkins, K. (eds) (2004) *Supervision as Collaboration in the Human Services. Building a Learning Culture*, London: Sage.

Avis, J. (2005) 'Beyond performativity: reflections on activist professionalism and the labour process in further education', *Journal of Education Policy*, 20(2): 209–22.

Ball, S. (2003) 'The teacher's soul and the terrors of performativity', *Journal of Education Policy*, 18(2): 215–28.

Beddoe, L. (2010) 'Surveillance or reflection: professional supervision in "the risk society"', *British Journal of Social Work*, 40: 1279–96.

Bogo, M., Gioberman, J. and Sussman, T. (2004) 'The field instructor as group worker: managing trust and competition in group supervision', *Journal of Social Work Education*, 40(1): 13–26.

Bolman, L. and Deal, T. (1997) *Reframing Organizations. Artistry, Choice and Leadership* (2nd edn) San Francisco: Jossey-Bass.

Bond, M. and Holland, S. (1998) *Skills of Clinical Supervision for Nurses: A Practical Guide for Supervisees, Clinical Supervisors and Managers*, Buckingham: Open University Press.

Bradley, G. and Höjer, S. (2009) 'Supervision reviewed: reflections on two different social work models in England and Sweden', *European Journal of Social Work*, 12(1): 71–85.

Brown, A. and Bourne, I. (1996) *The Social Work Supervisor*, Buckingham: Open University Press.

Butterworth, T. (1998) 'Clinical supervision as an emerging idea in nursing', in T. Butterworth, J. Faugier and P. Burnard (eds) *Clinical Supervision and Mentorship in Nursing*, Cornwall: Stanley Thornes Ltd, pp. 3–17.

Chaharbaghi, K. (2010) 'The audit dilemma in public services', *International Journal of Critical Accounting,* abstract accessed at www.uel.ac.uk/business/staff/kazemchaharbaghi.htm

Clough, R. (1995) 'Making supervision work in residential care', in J. Pritchard (ed.) *Good Practice in Supervision, Statutory and Voluntary Organisations*, London: Jessica Kingsley, pp. 20–36.

CWDC (2007) 'Providing effective supervision', accessed at www.cwdcouncil.org.uk/assets/0000/2832/Providing_Effective_Supervision_unit.pdf. Accessed 24.02.11.

Dahlberg, G., Moss, P. and Pence, A. (2007) *Beyond Quality in Early Childhood Education and Care* (2nd edn) London: Routledge.

Davies, B. (2003) 'Death to critique and dissent? The policies and practices of new managerialism and of "evidence-based practice"', *Gender and Education*, 15(1): 91–103.

Doel, M. and Sawdon, C. (1999) *The Essential Groupworker*, London: Jessica Kingsley.

Evans, L. (2008) 'Professionalism, professionality and the development of education professionals', *British Journal of Educational Studies*, 56(1): 20–38.

Everitt, A. and Hardiker, P. (1996) *Evaluating for Good Practice*, Basingstoke: Macmillan Press.

Evetts, J. (2005) 'The management of professionalism: a contemporary paradox', Conference paper presented at the 'Changing Teacher Roles, Identities and Professionalism' conference, October.

——(2006) 'Trust and professionalism: challenges and occupational changes', *Current Sociology*, 54(4): 515–531.

Hair, H. and O'Donoghue, K. (2009) 'Culturally relevant, socially just social work supervision: becoming visible through a social constructionist lens', *Journal of Ethnic and Cultural Diversity in Social Work*, 18: 70–88.

Hawkins, P. and Shohet, R. (2006) *Supervision in the Helping Professions* (3rd edn) Berkshire: Open University Press.

Hyrkas, K. and Appelqvist-Schmidlechner, K. (2003) 'Team supervision in multiprofessional teams: team members' descriptions of the effects as highlighted by group interviews', *Journal of Clinical Nursing*, 12: 188–97.

Ingram, G. and Harris, J. (2001) *Delivering Good Youth Work: A Working Guide to Surviving and Thriving*, Lyme Regis: Russell House Publishing.

Inskipp, F. and Proctor, B. (1993) *Making the Most of Supervision, Parts 1 and 2*, London: Cascade Publications.

Janis, I. (1972) *Victims of Groupthink*, Boston: Houghton Mifflin.

Johns, C. (2001) 'Depending on the intent and emphasis of the supervisor, clinical supervision can be a different experience', *Journal of Nursing Management*, 9(3): 139–45.

Kadushin, A. (1992) *Supervision in Social Work* (3rd edn) New York: Columbia University Press.

Kadushin, A. and Harkness, D. (2002) *Supervision in Social Work* (4th edn) New York and Chichester: Columbia University Press.

Kögler, H. (1999) *The Power of Dialogue: Critical Hermeneutics after Gadamer and Foucault*, Cambridge, MA: MIT Press.

Kuechler, C. (2006) 'Practitioners' voices: group supervisors reflect on their practice', *The Clinical Supervisor*, 25(1/2): 83–103.

Laird, J. (1998) 'Theorizing culture: narrative ideas and practice principles', in M. McGoldrick (ed.) *Re-visioning Family Therapy: Race, Culture, and Gender in Clinical Practice*, New York: Guilford Press, pp. 20–36.

Laming, H. (2003) *The Victoria Climbié Inquiry. Report of an Inquiry by Lord Laming*, CM 5730, London: The Stationery Office.

Marchant, H. (1987) 'Supervision: a training perspective', in M. Marken and M. Payne (eds) *Enabling and Ensuring Supervision in Practice* (2nd edn) Leicester: National Youth Bureau, pp. 35–44.

Marken, M. and Payne, M.(eds) (1987) *Enablng and Ensuring Supervision in Practice* (2nd edn) Leicester: National Youth Bureau.

O'Neill, O. (2002) *A Question of Trust*, Cambridge: Cambridge University Press.

Parton, N. (2003) 'Rethinking professional practice: the contributions of social constructionism and the feminist ethics of care', *British Journal of Social Work*, 33(1): 1–16.

Parton, N. and O'Byrne, P. (2000) *Constructive Social Work: Towards a New Practice*, London: Macmillan.

Payne, M. and Scott, T. (1982) 'Developing supervision of teams in field and residential social work – Part 1', Paper no.12, London: National Institute for Social Work.

Power, M. (1997) *The Audit Society: Rituals of Verification*, Oxford: Oxford University Press.

Preston-Shoot, M. (2007) *Effective Groupwork*, Basingstoke: Palgrave Macmillan.

Proctor, B. (2008) *Group Supervision: A Guide to Creative Practice* (2nd edn) London: Sage.

Sapin, K. (2009) *The Essential Skills for Youth Work Practice*, London: Sage.

Sawdon, C. and Sawdon, D. (1995) 'The supervision partnership', in J. Pritchard (ed.) *Good Practice in Supervision*, London: Jessica Kingsley, pp. 3–19.

Schön, D. (1987) *Educating the Reflective Practitioner*, San Francisco: Jossey-Bass.

Seden, J. and McCormick, M. (2011) 'Caring for yourself, being managed and professional development', in J. Seden, S. Matthews, M. McCormick and A. Morgan (eds) *Professional Development in Social Work: Complex Issues in Practice*, Abingdon: Routledge, pp. 171–77.

Senge, P. (1994) *The Fifth Discipline Fieldbook: Strategies and Tools for Building a Learning Organization*, New York: Doubleday.

Smith, C. (2001) 'Trust and confidence: possibilities for social work in "high modernity"', *British Journal of Social Work*, 31: 287–305.

Smith, M. (2005) 'The functions of supervision', *The Encyclopedia of Informal Education*. Accessed at www.infed.org.uk on 21.02.11

Tash, M. J. (1967) *Supervision in Youth Work*, London: London Council of Social Service, Reprinted by the YMCA National College 1984, 2000.

Taylor, C. and White, S. (2000) *Practising Reflexivity in Health and Welfare: Making Knowledge*, Buckingham: Open University Press.

Tegg, C. (1990) *The Uses of Supervision in Community Work: Talking Point no. 116*, Newcastle-upon-Tyne: Association of Community Workers.

Thompson, N. (1997) *Anti-discriminatory Practice* (2nd edn) Basingstoke: Macmillan.

Tsui, M. (1997) 'The roots of social work supervision: an historical review', *The Clinical Supervisor*, 15: 191–98.

Walker, S. (2001) 'Tracing the contours of postmodern social work', *British Journal of Social Work*, 31: 29–39.

Wilkerton, K. (2006) 'Peer supervision for the professional development of school counselors: toward an understanding of terms and findings', *Counselor Education and Supervision*, 46: 59–67.

Zorga, S., Dekleva, B. and Kobolt, A. (2001) 'The process of internal evaluation as a tool for improving peer supervision', *International Journal for the Advancement of Counselling*, 23: 151–62.

# 9 Managing centre-based youth work

## Jon Ord, with Mohamed Moustakim and Emily Wood

In this chapter we examine the role of the youth centre manager in the changing landscape of youth service provision. The chapter brings into sharp focus the dilemmas faced by many youth work managers in their attempts to reconcile the values, principles and practices of youth work with the culture of managerialism which has shaped many aspects of management and leadership of youth service provision in recent years.

The chapter begins with the historical development of centre-based youth provision, highlighting the impact of post-welfarism (Gewirtz, 2002) on centre-based youth work. In this respect, the changing roles and responsibilities of the youth centre manager will be critically examined, particularly in relation to managing buildings and managing provision. This is followed by an analysis of the community context of youth work, and finishes with an attempt to describe the future of youth centre management, at the heart of which is the need to resolve the value conflicts resulting from managing youth work provision within a managerialist culture.

### Changing times

The historical landscape of youth work is characterized by political and economic tensions at the root of which power and control persistently mediate the relationship between the state and young people (Davies, 2005). Although the beginnings of youth work in Britain can be traced back to the Sunday schools in the late eighteenth century and the ragged schools at the beginning of the nineteenth century, centre-based youth work began with the birth of the YMCA in London in 1844, and the youth institutes and clubs set up by Arthur Sweetman in the 1850s (Davies, 1999).

The government took some interest in youth work during both World War I and World War II, and the birth of the statutory youth service arguably resulted from the 1944 Education Act. However, it was the 1960s that saw the most significant expansion of centre-based youth work. The Albemarle Report (ME, 1960) signified a landmark in the history of the youth service as it set in motion a ten-year development programme, which included an unprecedented £23 million on the youth centre construction projects culminating in the creation of more than 3,000 new buildings (Davies, 1999: 61).

The youth projects created as a result of the Albemarle Report were considered to be innovative at the time, but by the mid-1980s they began to seem out of step with the interests of young people (Jeffs and Smith, 2006). Some contemporary youth centres more accurately reflect the modern age: their interior design and fittings reflect the ubiquity and importance of information technology; some even benefit from music studios, gyms, dance studios and beauty rooms (Durham University and YMCA,

2010). In many however, including a good many of the original Albemarle centres, the resources are often limited to pool and table tennis, a television and some computer games, as well as perhaps a kitchen to cook in (Ord, 2011). Prior to the neoliberal and managerialist reforms described in earlier chapters, youth clubs were viewed as spaces for young people to 'hang out', make friends and take part in educational and recreational activities of their choice (Robertson, 2005). Arguably, youth workers still see them in this way, but changes are being enforced.

Whilst the immediate impact of these reforms was considerable in formal education (Tomlinson, 2001), youth workers enjoyed relative professional freedom. Davies points out that during the 1980s, the youth service 'remained peripheral to Thatcherite plans' (1999: 13). There were attempts to galvanize the potential contribution that the youth service could make to the attainment of the government priorities, by attempting to introduce a 'core curriculum' via three ministerial conferences (NYB, 1990; 1991; NYA, 1992), thereby attempting to establish a set of 'priority outcomes which the service should seek to provide' (Ord, 2004: 44). However, the fraught debates culminated in an agreement to produce locally agreed curricula (Ord, 2007: 4) and the youth service fell back into 'neglect' (Davies, 1999: 13).

Compared to what has been described as the Albemarle 'golden age' (Davies, 1999), this period saw a decrease in the take-up of youth provision, particularly in the upper age range, which has been attributed to the widely available and more sophisticated means of entertainment at the disposal of many young people. As Jeffs and Smith suggest: 'The irresistible rise of commercial providers, including the expansion of home entertainment and leisure centres, has left the youth work sector a bit part player within an arena where once it was a central figure' (Jeffs and Smith, 2006: 27).

The renewed interest from New Labour in youth work was perhaps cautiously welcomed by many, as support for a struggling service was much needed. However, these policies have redefined the role of practitioners in fundamental ways. Bradford (2005) suggests that as a result of *Transforming Youth Work* (DfES, 2001; 2002) traditional expressive purposes of youth work have given way to instrumental ones. This has changed the focus of youth work from a collective political concern for the common good of society to economically driven goals couched in market-derived vocabulary, such as 'accountability, efficiency, effectiveness, value for money, cost control, customer satisfaction, service delivery, planning unit and quality assurance' (Matheson and Matheson, 2000: 67). Inevitably, these changes have had a significant impact on all aspects of the management of centre-based youth work, from the targeting of young people to managing buildings and the achievement of externally imposed targets.

## Targeting

Whilst youth work has perhaps always had some concern for what were historically referred to as the 'unattached' or the 'disaffected', New Labour accentuated this considerably. There is a danger of youth work becoming a service targeted at what are deemed to be 'problematic' young people, and of it losing its universal ethos (NYA, 2010; Davies, 2010). New Labour policies have specifically linked youth work delivery to young people deemed to be 'at risk' or Not in Education, Employment or Training (NEET) (DfES, 2001; 2002), as well as to a raft of other social problems such as teenage pregnancy, drug and alcohol misuse, and criminality (DfCSF, 2007; 2009).

This not only pathologizes young people and their issues, but is derived from ideological representations of young people as dysfunctional and in urgent need of expert intervention to return them to normality (Bradford, 2005). Young people are therefore 'constructed' as deficient perpetrators (Griffin, 1993) or thugs, users or victims (Jeffs and Smith, 1999). Implicit within these notions is the assumption that specialist intervention will help them regain self-esteem and put them on the 'straight and narrow'.

There is now an evident tension between universal and targeted provision which youth centre managers must balance. No doubt many are resisting the shift in priority towards only working with certain young people separated into groups, identified by their 'issues' (such as those at risk of engaging in criminal activity, becoming pregnant or misusing drugs). It would appear that youth centre managers are attempting to continue to provide sessions which are 'open access', but there is increasing pressure to provide closed group programmes, such as the Youth Inclusion Programmes (YIPs) or Young Mums/Dads courses (e.g. one afternoon a week for 10 weeks). Whilst it is acknowledged that these programmes can be beneficial for young people, it is argued they work best when integrated into an existing universal service. In this way some young people can be given the specialist support when needed and all young people benefit from building sustained relationships with both their peers and with youth workers in the informal setting of a youth centre. The targeted and universal dual provision also allows and encourages varied groups of young people to interact, enriching their diversity of experiences, enhancing community cohesion and cultural awareness. An example of this is at a youth centre in South London which provides and seeks to integrate the universal groups with the different targeted groups it works with, such as offenders, young dads and young Muslim women. This not only limits the 'pathologizing' of young people, as they are primarily seen as 'young people' not defined by a particular grouping, but ensures that young people are not just 'dumped' at the end of the programme, and left unsupported.

Another pressure on youth workers to provide short, closed programmes or courses, is the impact of targets. Whilst more will be said later about the impact of accreditation, it is important to make the link here between the pressure to meet accreditation targets and the proliferation of programmes which can be accredited. Youth workers are unlikely to meet their targets unless they provide a significant number of additional accreditation programmes for young people, whether that be through sport, music production, web design, or drama.

Where there is increasing focus on projects geared towards specific interventions, and issues, and which are time specific, there is a danger that there is too much focus on negative 'problems'. This type of provision is likely to change the relationship youth workers have with young people to a 'delivery and case work' model (Smith, 2003); and is not based on the expressed needs of young people, nor does 'it start where they are at' (Davies, 2005). To avoid this scenario it is important that a universal element of provision is retained.

Another implication of targeting of young people has been a narrowing of the designated age range to 13–19, which brings the traditional focus of youth centres into stark contrast. Whilst youth workers themselves have not traditionally worked with children under eight, prior to 2002 and the stipulations of Transforming Youth Work, youth centres would have catered for 8–11-year-olds in junior clubs and 11–13-year-olds in what were often described as intermediate clubs, as well as over 19s. The emphasis on 13–19-year-olds undermined the community context. They were no longer youth 'and community' centres with a remit for developing work across a broad age range, perhaps with preschools in the morning, and providing for a wide range of children and young people, as well as for older members of the community who might use the building to hold private functions, or host their own sports or social clubs; not to mention young adults, who still require support.

## Managing buildings

The management of the building is an integral part of the youth centre manager's role. The centre is a resource in itself, in that it provides a safe space for young people and enables a range of activities from sports, arts, cookery, and music to specific events.

### *Young people's ownership?*

Whether the building is designated as a 'youth centre', a 'youth and community centre' or a 'community centre' is significant. It would be a mistake to think that these are interchangeable and that the specific moniker does not have important implications. A community centre denotes a community and neighbourhood focus, and young people are very often not equal members of that community with equal rights as adults. A youth and community centre denotes a building that is used by all members of the community, including young people, taking part in a wide range of social, educational and recreational activities, which might include preschool, youth work and provision for the elderly. However, it is important who manages such a centre, and whose interests it serves. Too often both 'community centres' and 'youth and community centres' are dominated by the interests of adults. There can be benefits in sharing spaces, resulting in what is often termed intergenerational work. However, the prevailing situation is often one in which young people are being provisionally 'allowed' into an adult space, and continues the assumption that the young people need to learn from the adults.

Given the balance of power is in favour of the adults, and young people could arguably be described as an 'oppressed group' (Stein and Frost, 1992), it would be more beneficial for adults to share the young people's space, so that the adult community can learn about, and from, the young people. This would be more likely to improve community relations, and work toward tipping the balance of power around ownership of space.

Only a youth centre is primarily geared towards the needs and interests of young people: 'a space of their own, something which is rarely available to young people in other contexts' (Williamson, 1997: 180). The majority of public and private spaces that young people inhabit are essentially 'adult' spaces, including schools, the home, shopping centres, even the street, and local parks. Youth centres are the only spaces that are just for young people, and should be decorated and designed with, and for, them. Only within a designated 'youth space' can young people develop a sense of ownership, and begin to foster a sense of the 'club' which was at the heart of the original Albemarle ethos (ME, 1960). An ethos which continues, as Holman found: 'above all what came over was the importance of the club to young people, both as a place of refuge and safety, but also as the place where they made relationships with adults on an equal footing' (cited in Robertson, 2005: 53).

### The involvement of young people

It is important to involve young people in creating an inclusive, accessible and welcoming environment. Involvement in *making decisions* about the interior design and layout of the youth centre can provide valuable opportunities for young people to begin to develop a sense of ownership. But it is much more than this; participation and decision-making are not just about young people 'designing' or 'decorating' a centre. It ought to involve the young people in fundraising, allocating resources, deciding on and creating activities, evaluating and developing the services they receive, and having a voice in issues which concern them and their communities. However, participation and its resulting 'empowerment', if it is to be anything other than a mere 'buzzword' (Thomson 2006: 21), 'is ultimately about power' (Ord, 2007: 47).

The extent therefore to which these essential participative practices can be developed is dependent upon the manager's ownership and control of the centre, and the extent to which young people's interests are central within the management of that centre, as well as within the wider organization or service. Participative practices in reality are often restricted. For example, the adults involved in a playgroup that uses the youth centre during the day may find it objectionable to have posters about drugs on the walls and insist on their removal. Financial controls potentially limit the ability of youth centre managers to delegate, and limits to participation in decision-making can also be imposed by structural and organizational arrangements, such as contracting of services. Health and safety demands may also limit young people getting involved in activities such as painting and decorating the centre. Participation ought to be aimed at encouraging young people to take control and become young leaders in our youth centres (see Baker, 1996), as is articulated through the various participation ladders (Hart, 1992; Huskins, 1996).

Importantly, as alluded to above, the extent to which young people actually have the power to make, and influence, decisions is at the heart of meaningful involvement. However, given managerialism leans towards the micromanagement and control of workers it is hard to imagine that the empowerment of young people is going to be fully embraced. Youth centre managers can therefore find themselves caught in the middle between the requests made by young people, and the organizational constraints. Too often youth centre managers' attempts to work participatively are thwarted by the many restrictions placed on the empowerment of young people.

### Democratic management

Arguably 'full-time workers spend too much time talking to each other and not enough time working with young people, part-timers, and community groups' (Jeffs and Smith, 1988: 246). If the commitments to young people as partners in learning and decision-making, and to helping them to develop their own sets of values, are to be realized in youth work, they must not only permeate the relationships between youth workers and young people, but amongst the staff as well. A team effort or distributed leadership is therefore essential to fulfil organizational goals (Lashway, 2003), particularly given the multi-faceted nature of youth work, where involvement in collaborative decision-making is not only consistent with a youth work ethos, it also promotes high staff morale, greater sense of ownership and intrinsic motivation to improve practice. This can only be achieved if youth centre managers treat their colleagues fairly and equitably. As we saw earlier in Chapter 3, from a humanist perspective, a concern for the wellbeing of staff often leads to an improvement in the commitment and motivation of workers. Fullan rightly suggests, 'a leader who does not treat others well and fairly will be a leader without followers' (2004: 11). It is argued that a shared vision can only be genuinely facilitated by a democratic style of leadership. Whether it be with the design and use of recording and evaluation forms, feedback on possible new strategies and ways of working, or the ways in which young people's challenging behaviour is dealt with, the involvement of staff and a team approach will reap dividends in both the short and long term.

### Maintenance

Robertson (2005) identified a problem with refurbishment of youth centres with the original Albemarle project. Whilst considerable capital expenditure was provided for the construction of a significant number of youth centres, no facility was provided for ongoing refurbishment and expenditure on improvements. This situation, for many centres, continues to this day, where funding for maintenance, refurbishment and development remains an issue. This is evidenced by recent research (Ord, 2011) which demonstrated consistent underinvestment in the fifty-year history of youth centre development in the Royal Borough of Kingston.

It is difficult to generalize about the mechanisms through which maintenance and refurbishment are managed. Some youth centres will have delegated controllable expenditure in their allocated budgets, which is limited to the purchase of consumables but does not extend to building repairs and maintenance, which are controlled centrally by the local authority. In such situations, one can see evidence of the managerialist legacy of 'best value' and 'compulsory competitive tendering' as the most economic solution is sought. However, the process of involving local authority contractors does not necessarily ensure the job is done either efficiently or cheaply, as it has been found that simple jobs could have been done much more quickly if local tradesmen had been used. Neither in reality does the supplier necessarily provide the best service, and this procurement process limits the responsiveness of the centre manager. At the other extreme, perhaps more common in the voluntary sector, the youth centre manager will be responsible for organizing all aspects of maintenance and refurbishment.

### Health and safety

The rise of managerialism and the re-emphasis on the importance of managerial controls, and stringent mechanistic procedures, has seen an increase in concerns with health and safety. Whilst clearly youth centre managers must maintain a proper concern for both the 'health' and 'safety' of all who use the centre, arguably the bureaucratization of health and safety, and the culture of fear which underlies it, has had a negative impact on youth work delivery. Local authorities are no doubt the worst culprits when it comes to overbearing health and safety policies, as documented by Pearce (2007; 2009). But the voluntary sector is not immune either. Although admittedly the examples Pearce cites are not from youth work, they provide clear evidence of the absurdity of health and safety regulations. Examples range from young people being banned from removing their long sleeved sweatshirts during PE unless they have written permission from their parents (to prevent sunburn), to the removal of a hundred mature yew trees from a children's playground for fear of the children being poisoned by eating their leaves or berries (2007: 109), as well as blanket bans on school trips and out-ings (2007: 22), and even a school which banned conkers for fear of a nut allergy (2007: 38).

Such 'crazy' applications of health and safety guidelines fail to acknowledge an important distinction between 'theoretical risks' and 'serious, genuine or practical concerns'. Health and safety ought to be concerned with the latter; it is neither prac-ticable, nor possible, to minimize theoretical risks. Whilst perhaps youth work is not guilty of the worst excesses of health and safety regulations, it is naive to think they are immune from the 'culture of fear' and 'risk aversion' which underpin them. One example of how this has permeated the culture of youth work is in the widespread acceptance that a youth worker cannot give a young person a condom unless they have undertaken specific training and certification. This is often regarded as completely unproblematic, it being argued that training is widely available, and often at least one youth worker at the centre has undertaken such training. However whilst no doubt training can improve one's understanding of the issues underlying safe sex and contra-ception, the implication of such regulations is that a youth worker is a danger to young people unless they have undergone such training. Preventing youth workers from handing out condoms until they have undergone training is a misuse of health and safety concerns and a bureaucratization of, and an unnecessary attempt to control, risk.

Perhaps the most obvious way that onerous health and safety regulations have impacted on youth work is through risk assessments. Whilst clearly it is important for any manager to adequately assess genuine risks to young people undertaking activities in and around the centre, as well as on trips and outings, risk assessments are having a detrimental effect on practice and bureaucratizing youth work. For example, one county council youth service had an inordinate number of risk assessments at its youth centres, covering such 'inherently dangerous' tasks as: 'emptying bins', 'running the tuck shop', 'playing a game of rounders' and 'putting up displays'. The bureaucracy of risk assessments is also having a negative effect on the spontaneity of youth work. Many youth workers now feel they can't just leave the centre and go to the local park in the evening, without adequate risk assessment. Youth work practice is littered with examples where the fluidity and responsiveness of youth work is negatively impacted upon by the restrictions imposed by risk assessments, a recent example of which was the inability of youth workers to call into the local shop or take-away on the way back from a trip because it wasn't on the risk assessment.

Risk assessments do not need to be interpreted as the micromanagement of theore-tical risks. The Health and Safety Executive's guidance on 'sensible' risk assessments states that they should focus on: 'balancing benefits and risks, with a focus on reducing real risks' HSE (2011). Equally importantly, the HSE maintains that:

> Sensible risk management *is not* about:
>
> Creating a totally risk free society
> Generating useless paperwork mountains
> Scaring people by exaggerating or publicising trivial risks
> Stopping important recreational and learning activities for individuals where the risks are managed.
>
> (HSE, 2011)

Risk assessments can also be 'dynamic', that is they can be done in real time: 'Focusing attention on the unfolding risks which may emerge as relevant circumstances change' (Hartley, 2009: 153). It is incumbent on the youth centre manager therefore to critically evaluate the current culture of health and safety and instigate more realistic guidelines which embrace the fluidity and responsiveness of youth work practice.

### The nightmare scenario for youth work managers

It is evident that the demands upon youth centre managers are ever increasing. Bamber (2000) describes this as the nightmare scenario (see Figure 9.1 below): a situation in which the youth centre manager is torn between an ever increasing number of competing priorities, which include the need to supervise staff, obtain funding, devise policies, network with other agencies, etc.

Importantly. Bamber notes that this situation significantly restricts the amount of face-to-face work that youth centre managers can deliver: 'where the face-to-face practitioners of yesteryear have become the managers of youth work today' (2000: 5). Bamber notes that this situation is exacerbated by excessive managerialism, and ironically this

> Frustrate[s] the recent policy initiatives concerning lifelong learning, social exclusion and active citizenship because the realisation of these initiatives requires the face-to-face commitment of highly trained professional educators.
>
> (2000: 5)

Youth centre managers' expertise is in youth work and arguably they should be spending a significant proportion of their time with young people and with other workers, who can learn from them.

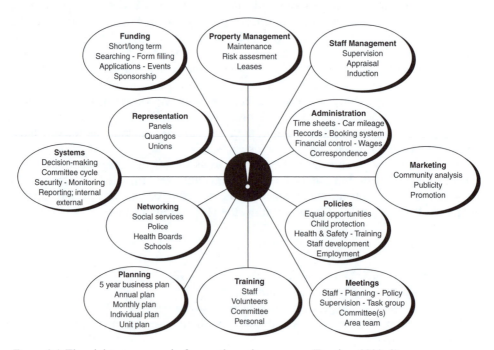

*Figure 9.1* The nightmare scenario for youth work managers (Bamber, 2000: 9)

## Managing delivery

### *Targets*

One of the most obvious and detrimental ways in which managerialism has impacted on youth centre management has been in the form of targets introduced by Transforming Youth Work (DfES, 2002). These ranged from the number of young people the service is in 'contact' with, 'participation' (the number of personal and social development opportunities offered to young people), 'recorded outcomes' and the most contentious of all 'accredited outcomes' (DfES, 2002: 16–17).

In many ways the introduction of the Transforming Youth Work targets represents the culmination of a process of increased instrumentalism in youth work previously identified by amongst others Davies (1986), Jeffs and Smith (1994), and Bradford (2000). Whilst this instrumental approach had a more general theme of control, the Transforming Youth Work targets had a much more specific focus geared towards 'maximising employability'. Confirmation of this can be found in the guidance on accreditation published by the NYA, where the criteria for accreditation requires it to: 'have currency/ credibility outside youth work … and where possible, a link to employment, education or training' (Flint, 2005: 6). The impact on youth work of recorded, and accredited outcomes was ensured, when in 2003 they became the official means by which local authority's youth services were to be made accountable, when the Transforming Youth Work targets were adopted as the best value performance indicators (BVPI 221a, 221b).

As a result an instrumental ideology has come to dominate youth work which results in the adoption of youth work approaches which valorize the acquisition of skills preparing young people for the world of work, over the development of autonomy and critical inquiry. Giroux cogently expressed this when he said:

> The pedagogy of critical inquiry and ethical understanding has given way to the logic of instrumental reason, with its directed focus on the learning of discrete competencies and basic skills.
>
> (1983: 43)

It has been argued that accreditation has a detrimental effect on youth work practice (Smith, 2003; Ord, 2007; Lehal, 2010), suggesting it formalizes practice and converts the process of youth work from one which 'starts where young people are at' to one which is driven by the requirements of an accreditation syllabus. There are youth workers who claim that they have not altered their practice and have merely accredited existing work that is undertaken by young people within their centre. Examples of this, however, often focus on work which is more easily accredited, such as music or outdoor education projects, where particular skills are learnt. Some would argue accreditation itself is not incompatible with good quality youth work, but setting targets inevitably skews provision. Evidence is emerging of how youth workers are struggling with the demands of accreditation and how it is impacting on their practice. Examples exist of youth centres which have around 250 young people attending during the year, being given an accreditation target of 150. Inevitably as a result, Lehal notes, projects 'which don't lead to accreditation but they lead to young people gaining an awful lot, are being squeezed out' (2010: 100).

An indication of how managerialist practices have become embedded within youth work management, is confirmed by the response to the abolition of the best value performance indicators (BVPIs) the youth work targets. That the iron grip of managerialism had been loosened slightly was not greeted with joy and celebration. On the contrary, youth service senior managers have in the main, retained a commitment to these targets (Davies and Merton, 2009) and in some instances not even informed youth workers that there is no longer an obligation to accredit their work with young people.

*Programming*

In addition to the obvious impact of targets on the delivery of centre-based youth work, of equal importance has been the shift to programmed work. As we saw previously, this predated New Labour, with the partially successful attempts to impose a curriculum on youth work in the late 1980s and early 1990s (NYB, 1990; 1991; NYA,1992). Although youth work did not have a set curriculum imposed upon it, it did have to begin to articulate its educational practice in terms of a curriculum, which has the potential to undermine the process approach to youth work (Ord, 2004, 2007). With Transforming Youth Work, renewed attempts were made to impose a set curriculum (DfES, 2002; Merton and Wylie, 2002). Whilst the impact of this new curriculum appears minimal (Ord, 2007), of more importance has been the emphasis on youth work 'programmes'.

As we saw in Chapter 6 in the discussion on planning, it is important that youth workers are proactive in the 'informal education' of young people. However, ensuring youth workers plan specific programmes which lead to quantifiable and measurable outcomes undermines the informal and convivial nature of youth work (Smith, 2003). Nowadays youth centres are now much more likely to have projects in addition to, and perhaps even instead of, open, generic youth clubs. Such projects will be geared towards learning specific skills or gaining increased knowledge, which ultimately can be recorded and accredited. This overemphasis on programming unnecessarily formalizes youth work.

## Managing the community context

Whether or not the building is designated as a 'youth centre', 'community centre' or 'youth and community centre', there is always a community context to the youth work which is undertaken in and around that building. Traditionally youth work has appreciated the importance of this community context, and the youth centre manager would be located at the heart of the community. This would often have been formalized through the establishment of local management or advisory committees for the centres. Jeffs and Smith identified the beginnings of the demise of these commitments in 1988 when they observed: 'some authorities have attempted to dispense with the services of local management or advisory committees' (1988: 246), noting that this was: 'a further expression of centralism and technicism' (ibid.). By the new millennium this process could well have been complete, as Ord's research into youth centres in one London borough demonstrates that the last management committee was abolished in 2003 (Ord, 2011). Even in the voluntary sector, which in theory has more reliance on a committee structure, as is demonstrated in Chapter 13, trustees of voluntary organizations and the resulting committees are increasingly removed from their community base. The context for community engagement in youth work is now more likely to be within local 'Safer Neighbourhood Teams' and in work with Police Community Support Officers (PCSOs).

Jeffs and Smith (1988) note that youth workers themselves may well have colluded with this process, perhaps thinking that it is an affront to their professionalism and resenting that 'amateurs' have power over them and their work. However, the demise of such committees represents a gradual abstraction of the youth centre manager from the community, which represents a significant loss to the potential of the youth (and community) work. Lacey (1987) reminds us that working in a community-based building means we are inevitably working with adults as well as young people, whether that be with parents, other adult users of the building or local residents. Whilst she acknowledges this is time-consuming she also rightly points out that there are significant benefits of an inclusive approach to the wider community. These benefits are both for young people, as they are more likely to be accepted as part of the community as a youth worker advocates on their behalf, and also for the members of the wider community as they take an active interest in the centre.

Lacey argues that there is much more similarity between community work and youth work than is often acknowledged. She draws on the Fairbairn-Milson report, which recommended that: 'the youth and community service must recognize the adult status of those clients drawn from the upper age range who must be encouraged to play an active part' (1987: 39). Indeed, some of those who do get involved with the centre may well end up as future workers. This process of 'growing your own' is an essential aspect of a vibrant centre and is well documented by Rogers and Smith's collection of essays (2010). For example, Hill makes the point that: 'Effective youth work with young people does not happen in isolation ... it is vital that young people are part of a community ... and it is also vital that there is a community support' (Hill, 2010: 104), whilst McLaughlin et al. 'found that locally grown youth work tends to have a better understanding of the needs of the area, is able to be responsive to local concerns and more highly regarded by those who use its services' (cited in Jolly, 2010: 8).

The apparent separation between youth work's emphasis on young people and community work's focus on adults is further questioned by the work of Stein in Minnesota, USA. He challenges the isolation and abstraction of youth work from its community base, through the project: 'Learning Dreams'. The premise of his work is to harness the aspirations of parents on the basis that this will in turn influence the aspirations of their children: 'We need a program like Learning Dreams to get parents excited and help parents accomplish their own dreams so that they can help their children reach their dreams' (Learning Dreams, 2011).

Recent youth policy has exacerbated the alienation of young people from their communities. The liberal and unnecessary use of ASBOs, curfews and the use of mosquito devices restricts young people's ability to move and meet freely within their community. A narrowing of the age range of youth work to 13–19 has further undermined the community context of youth work. Youth centre managers must reassert the importance of the community context. Post-welfarism has brought about a distinct shift in terms of accountability, and this is no less noticeable within youth centre management. Youth work accountability is no longer framed around a notion of youth workers being located at the heart of communities (Smith, 1994; Jeffs and Smith, 2005) and being directly accountable to both the young people and their communities. But in line with other public servants, youth workers have latterly become accountable to bureaucrats, regulators and politicians, thereby changing the relationship between the state and its citizens from a political commitment to economic transaction (Biesta, 2004).

## The future of youth centre management

Given the evident incongruity of youth work principles with managerialist approaches to managing centre-based youth provision, many youth workers find themselves in what McNiff and Whitehead (2006) describe as a 'living contradiction'. This is due to the realization that their values are denied in their practice by institutional constraints. For example, working towards externally imposed targets undermines a youth centre manager's attempts to work participatively, and democratically. As a result youth centre managers are likely to experience a discrepancy between their attitudes and their behaviour, or what social psychologists have described as 'cognitive dissonance' (Festinger, 1957; Aronson, 1968; Steele, 1988; Elliot and Devine, 1994).

Such cognitive dissonance, where people find themselves in situations where their behaviour conflicts with their attitudes, is difficult to resolve. Workers and managers would need to either change their behaviour or change attitudes. However, changing their behaviour would involve refusing to respond to what would be described as legitimate requests from an employer, and might lead to disciplinary action. On the other hand, following the path of least resistance by changing their attitudes to accommodate the unacceptable expectations will necessarily involve a degree of rationalization, and going against both personal and professional values. It would certainly appear that the time is right to mobilize action in support of fundamental youth work values and their resulting practices. But it should be remembered of course that challenging is time-consuming, exhausting and often frustrating, and one can sympathize with youth centre managers who take the line of least resistance. As we saw in Chapter 4, resistance is not something which ought to be just 'managed out' but is a healthy part of a democratic process which ought to be at the heart of good management. The voice of youth workers is being mobilized through campaigns such as In Defence of Youth Work (IDYW, 2011), and managers must listen to the valid concerns of practitioners.

The future of youth centre management, at the time of writing, is in considerable flux. The unprecedented cuts are likely to have considerable impact upon not only how centres are managed, but whether those centres continue to exist. The latest predictions are that: 'Up to 3,000 local authority youth workers face losing their jobs by April 2012 as youth services grapple with average budget cuts of 28 per cent in the next financial year' (Hillier, 2011). Whilst in some instances face-to-face work and youth centres are being protected, as the tiers of middle management face the brunt of the cuts, this is by no means always the case.

The priority of retaining face-to-face work is evidently focused upon targeted youth work, as a study by CHYPS revealed: 'The services most affected will be open-access youth clubs and centres ... Ninety-six per cent of the 41 heads of youth services that responded said these would either be reduced or stopped altogether by April 2012' (Hillier, 2011); a situation not helped by a recent statement by the head of the National Youth Agency which appeared to formally embrace a commitment to the continuation of targeted work and the demise of open access, universal provision (Davies, 2010; NYA, 2010). In such situations where targeted youth work is overwhelmingly prioritized, youth workers are expected to deliver short programmes, to act as signposts, or undertake one-to-one support. There are also cases where the name 'youth worker' is being changed to 'key worker' or 'triage worker'. The danger here is as Glover points out: 'developing targeted work at the expense of the universal offer leaves the whole service vulnerable' (2010: 9). Even where individual youth centres are not facing immediate closure the example set by Manchester City Council is not uncommon, where: 'the council has decided to outsource many of its youth services, including youth centres' (Mahadevan, 2011). The cuts programme will undoubtedly accelerate the process of commissioning of youth services, and in particular youth centres.

Despite these gloomy prospects facing youth centres across the country, ironically there is a new development which is in stark contrast. The Myplace initiative arising out of New Labour's *Aiming High for Young People: A 10 Year Strategy for Positive Activities* (DfCSF, 2007) has provided funding for a significant number of 'world-class youth facilities' (Durham University and YMCA, 2010). In the region of £272 million has been made available to construct around seventy youth centres (ibid.). These centres have an impressive array of high quality sports, dance and drama facilities, as well as music studios, media production, and cybercafés (ibid.).

Myplace is not without its critics. Fogg argues: 'Little has been said about whether this is truly the best way to spend this money … [maintaining] the scheme will do little to upgrade the aging youth facilities in our towns and villages' (2009: 9), suggesting that it would have been better to allocate the money to local authorities to both improve existing facilities and have the time to invest the money appropriately, as it is alleged that the Myplace timescale did not appreciate the 'problems with finding sites and securing planning permission' (ibid.).

Although these criticisms might have some validity, it is perhaps a little churlish to complain about the first government initiative since Albemarle fifty years ago, which provided capital expenditure for the construction of new youth centres. It is hoped that Glover is right, and if we: 'make them a success … more will follow' (2010: 9).

## Conclusion

For the youth centres that survive this turbulent time, whether they are retained within the local authority or, as appears more likely, commissioned out to the voluntary sector, it is arguably time to take stock, and reassess the impact of managerialism on youth centre management. Difficulties and dilemmas in reconciling and balancing managerialist demands and expectations have been shown to be at odds with the core values of youth work. Youth work managers are in a position in which they can begin to challenge the managerialist practices which are at odds with their beliefs, and those of the youth workers and of the young people. We would argue for the return of democracy to the heart of youth centres, and to their management, as well as a re-establishment of the community context to youth work practice delivered in these centres.

## Questions for reflection and discussion

1   In what ways has the community context been eroded from youth centre management, and what can be done to reinstate this valuable aspect of youth work?
2   How can young people's involvement in both the delivery and management of youth work be maximized?
3   How can the management of the youth centre become more democratic?
4   What is the role of the youth centre in twenty-first-century youth work, how is it changing, and what can be done to ensure that it best meets the needs of young people?

## Further reading

Baker, J. (1996) *The Fourth Partner: Participant or Consumer?* Leicester: Youth Work Press.

Bamber, J. (2000) 'Managing youth work in Scotland: a diversionary tale', *Youth and Policy*, Summer, no. 68: 5–18.

Bradford, S. (2005) 'Modernising youth work: from the universal to the particular and back again', in Harrison, R. and Wise, C. (eds) *Working with Young People*, London: Sage, pp. 57–69.

Rogers, A. and Smith, M. K. (2010) *Journeying Together: Growing Youth Work and Youth Workers in Local Communities*, Lyme Regis: RHP.

## References

Aronson, E. (1968) 'Dissonance theory: progress and problems', in Abelson, R., Aronson, E., McGuire, W., Newcomb, T., Rosenberg, M. and Tannenbaum, P. (eds) *Theories of Cognitive Consistency: A Sourcebook*, Chicago: Rand-McNally, pp. 5–27.

Baker, J. (1996) *The Fourth Partner: Participant or Consumer?* Leicester: Youth Work Press.

Bamber, J. (2000) 'Managing youth work in Scotland: a diversionary tale', *Youth and Policy*, Summer, no. 68: 5–18.

Biesta, G. J. J. (2004) 'Education, accountability and the ethical demand: can the democratic potential of accountability be regained?' *Educational Theory*, 54(3): 233–50.

Bradford, S. (2000) 'Disciplining practices: new ways of making youth workers accountable', *International Journal of Adolescents and Youth*, vol. 9: 45–63.

——(2005) 'Modernising youth work: from the universal to the particular and back again', in Harrison, R. and Wise, C. (eds) *Working with Young People*, London: Sage, pp. 57–69.

Davies, B. (1986) *Threatening Youth: Towards a National Youth Policy*, Milton Keynes: Open University Press.

——(1999) *From Voluntaryism to Welfare State: A History of the Youth Service in England, Volume 1: 1939 – 1979*, Leicester: Youth Work Press.

——(2005) 'Threatening Youth revisited: youth policies under New Labour', *The Encyclopaedia of Informal Education*, www.infed.org/archives/bernard_davies/revisiting_threatening_youth.htm

——(2010) 'Open letter to the chief executive of the National Youth Agency', accessed as an attachment at www.cypnow.co.uk/news/1031676, dated 29 October.

Davies, B. and Merton, B. (2009) *Squaring the Circle? Findings of a 'Modest Inquiry' into the State of Youth Work Practice in a Changing Policy Environment*, Report, Leicester De Montfort University, available at www.dmu.ac.uk/Images/Squaring%20the%20Circle_tcm6-50166.pdf

DfCSF (2009) *Targeted Youth Support: Next Steps*, London: HMSO.

——(2007) *Targeted Youth Support: A Guide*, London: HMSO.

DfES (2001) *Transforming Youth Work: Developing Youth Work for Young People*, London: HMSO.

——(2002) *Transforming Youth Work: Resourcing Excellent Youth Services*, London: HMSO.

Durham University and YMCA, George Williams College (2010) *MyPlace Evaluation: Interim Report*. Available at: www.education.gov.uk/publications/RSG/AllRsgPublications/Page9/MYPLACE-INT-REP

Elliot, A. and Devine, P. (1994) 'On the motivational nature of cognitive dissonance: dissonance as psychological discomfort', *Journal of Personality and Social Psychology*, 67 (June): 382–94.

Farnham, D. and Horton, S. (eds) (1999) *Public Management in Britain*, London: Macmillan.

Festinger, L. (1957) *A Theory of Cognitive Dissonance*, Stanford, CA: Stanford University Press.

Flint, W. (2005) *Recording Young People's Progress and Accreditation in Youth Work*, Leicester: NYA.

Fogg, R. (2009) 'The Myplace fund is a missed opportunity', *Children and Young People Now*, 6 January, p. 9. www.cypnow.co.uk/news/871385/Myplace-fund-missed-opportunity/

Fullan, M. (2004) 'Leadership and sustainability', Hot Seat Paper, University of Toronto, Urban Leadership Community.

Gewirtz, S. (2002) *The Managerial School: Post-Welfarism and Social Justice in Education*, London: Routledge.

Giroux, H. (1983) *Theory and Resistance in Education*, Westport, CT: Bergin and Garvey.

Glover, G. (2010) 'Supercentres deliver super youth work', *Children and Young People Now*, 1 March, p. 9. www.cypnow.co.uk/news/985194/Super-centres-deliver-super-youth-work/

Griffin, C. (1993) *Representations of Youth: The Study of Youth and Adolescence in Britain and America*, Oxford: Polity Press.

Hart, R. (1992) *Children's Participation: From Tokenism to Citizenship, Innocenti Essays, no. 4*, Florence: UNICEF.

Hartley, H. (2009) *Sport, Physical Recreation and the Law*, Abingdon: Routledge

Hill, S. (2010) 'Creating and sustaining a philosophy for development', in Rogers, A. and Smith, M. K. (eds) *Journeying Together: Growing Youth Work and Youth Workers in Local Communities*, Lyme Regis: RHP, pp. 92–105.

Hillier, A. (2011) 'True scale of council youth service cuts revealed', *Youth Work Weekly*, 8 February. www.cypnow.co.uk/bulletins/Youth-Work-Weekly/news/1053491/?DCMP=EMC-Youth WorkWeekly

HSE (2011) 'Principles of sensible risk management', www.hse.gov.uk/risk/principlespoints.htm (accessed 23 March 2011).

Huskins, J. (1996) *Quality Work with Young People*, London: Youth Clubs UK.

IDYW (2011) In Defence of Youth Work Campaign. www.indefenceofyouthwork.org.uk/wordpress/ (accessed 25 March 2011).

Jeffs, T. and Smith, M. (1988) 'The promise of management for youth work', in Jeffs, T. and Smith, M. (eds) *Welfare and Youth Work Practice*, Basingstoke: Macmillan, pp. 230–51.

——(1994) 'Young people, youth work and a new authoritarianism', *Youth and Policy*, Autumn, no. 46: 17–32.

——(1999) 'The problem of "youth" for youth work', *Youth and Policy*, Winter, no. 62: 45–66.

——(2005) *Informal Education: Conversation, Democracy and Learning*, Nottingham: Education Heretics Press.

——(2006) 'Where is *Youth Matters* taking us?' *Youth and Policy*, Spring, no. 91: 23–39.

Jolly, J. (2010) 'Local youth work', in Rogers, A. and Smith, M. K. (eds) *Journeying Together: Growing Youth Work and Youth Workers in Local Communities*, Lyme Regis: RHP, pp. 1–12.

Lacey, F. (1987) 'Youth workers as community workers' in Jeffs, T. and Smith, M. (eds) *Youth Work*, Basingstoke: Macmillan, pp. 38–51.

Lashway, L. (2003) 'Distributed leadership', in *Clearing House on Educational Management (CEPM)*, College of Education, University of Oregon, Research Roundup 19, 4. Available at https://scholarsbank.uoregon.edu/xmlui/bitstream/handle/1794/3487/roundups_Summer_2003.pdf?sequence=1 (accessed 5 July 2011).

Learning Dreams (2011) www.learningdreams.org/ (accessed 24 March 2011).

Lehal, R. (2010) 'Targeting for youth workers', in Batsleer, J. and Davies, B. (eds) *What Is Youth Work?* Exeter: Learning Matters, pp. 90–103.

McNiff, J. and Whitehead, J. (2006) *Action Research: Living Theory*, London: Sage.

Mahadevan, J. (2011) 'Manchester to slash children's services budget by 26 per cent', *Children and Young People Now*, 8 February. www.cypnow.co.uk/bulletins/Daily-Bulletin/news/1053818/?DCMP=EMC-DailyBulletin (accessed 27 February 2011).

Matheson, C. and Matheson, D. (2000) *Educational Issues in the Learning Age*, London: Continuum.

Merton, B. and Wylie, T. (2002) *Towards a Contemporary Curriculum*, Leicester: NYA.

ME (1960) *Youth Service in England and Wales (Albemarle Report)*, London: HMSO/Ministry of Education.

NYA (1992) *Planning and Evaluation in a time of Change: The Next Step – report of the Third Ministerial Conference*, Leicester: NYA.

National Youth Agency (2001) *Ethical Conduct in Youth Work: A Statement of Values and Principles*, Leicester: NYA.

——(2010) *The National Youth Agency's Response to the Spending Review Framework*, http://swf.edocr.com/8b00127eed4eb91002c63afc831d678c8d71608c.swf (accessed 25 March 2011).

NYB (1990) *Danger or Opportunity: Towards a Core Curriculum for the Youth Service*, Leicester: NYB.

——(1991) *Towards a Core Curriculum for the Youth Service: The Next Step – report of the Second Ministerial Conference*, Leicester NYB.

Ord, J. (2004) 'Youth Work Curriculum and Transforming Youth Work agenda', *Youth and Policy*, Spring, no. 83: 43–59.

——(2007) *Youth Work: Process, Product and Practice: Creating an Authentic Curriculum in Work with Young People*, Lyme Regis: RHP.

——(2011) 'The provision of "Space and Place": The Mixed Blessing of the Albemarle Legacy for Kingston Youth Service', in *Reflecting the Past: Essays in the History of Youth and Community Work*, Lyme Regis: RHP, pp. 130–45.

Pearce, A. (2007) *Playing It Safe: The Crazy World of Britain's Health and Safety Regulations*, London: Friday Books.

——(2009) *It's Health and Safety Gone Mad! 1001 Crazy Safety 'Crimes'*, London: Gibson Square.

Robertson, S. (2005) *Youth Clubs: Association, Participation, Friendship and Fun*, Lyme Regis: RHP.

Rogers, A. and Smith, M. K. (2010) *Journeying Together: Growing Youth Work and Youth Workers in Local Communities*, Lyme Regis: RHP.

Smith, M. K. (1994) *Local Education: Community, Conversation, Praxis*, Buckingham: Open University Press.

——(2003) 'From the youth work to youth development', *Youth and Policy*, Spring, no. 79: 46–59.

Steele, C. (1988) 'The psychology of self-affirmation: sustaining the integrity of the self', in Berkowitz, L. (ed.) *Advances in Experimental Social Psychology*, vol. 21, New Jersey: Lawrence Erlbaum, pp. 261–302.

Stein, M. and Frost, N. (1992) 'Empowerment and child welfare', in Coleman, J. C. and Adamson, C. W. (eds) *Youth Policy in the 1990s: The Way Forward*, London: Routledge, pp. 161–71.

Thomson, N. (2006) *Empowerment*, Lyme Regis: RHP.

Tomlinson, S. (2001) *Education in a Post-Welfare Society*, Buckingham: Open University Press.

Williamson, H. (1997) 'The needs of young people aged 15 to 19 and the youth work response', in *Youth and Policy: Contexts and Consequences*, Aldershot: Ashgate.

# 10 Towards an 'intelligence based approach' to detached youth work management

## Graeme Tiffany

This chapter sets out to argue that our understanding of 'what detached youth work is' is critical to its management. The success of this practice is seen as dependent on a distinctive methodology. This, in turn, requires a particular form of management for it to develop and flourish.

### Current context of detached youth work

The reality of detached youth work today is characterised by a good deal of divergence from the traditional analytical model (Goetchius and Tash, 1967), whose work is invoked by Smith (2007) as offering hope and possibility to those 'imprisoned within a pseudo management discourse of delivery'.

A tale from colleagues in France perhaps illustrates this point as well as any from the UK. Those who have ventured there will no doubt have come across those large 'do-it-yourself' warehouses in almost every town and city, called 'Mr. Bricolage'. French detached youth workers now refer to themselves, with considerable irony, as the same (CNLAPS, 2008). Policy makers and managers, they argue, now see them as the ones to 'fix' almost any problem, just as the handyman character Mr. Bricolage is seen as being able to do. Needless to say they are incensed by this view of their role.

This context is all too familiar to those working in the UK. They have (especially in recent times) been increasingly co-opted and incorporated into myriad social policy agendas. These include alternative curriculum programmes, the Teenage Pregnancy Strategy, drug prevention projects and a wide range of crime prevention initiatives. As the name suggests, *Reconnecting Detached Youth Work* (Tiffany, 2007a) was an attempt to articulate a disconnection from the history of detached youth work as a socio-educational practice (Dynamo International, 2009: 25), grounded in a democratic tradition. A parallel culture of detached youth workers being tasked to solve social problems is much in evidence. Not that detached youth workers haven't always tried to alleviate the problems experienced by young people as part of their wider educational remit. The difference is that, these days, what constitutes a 'problem' is increasingly prescribed by policy. Little account is taken of whether these are the problems identified by young people themselves. Just as in France, detached youth work here seems to have morphed into a residual category in which a whole range of policy objectives have been handed over to these 'practitioners with access': those in contact with the young people with whom so many other agencies fail to engage.

Therein lies the problem. This 'catch-all' view of detached youth work is problematic in terms of detached work's ability to achieve good outcomes. This has the further, potentially more damaging impact: it invites a general form of management which, it will be argued, further undermines detached youth work. On the other hand, the use of a more precise definition of detached youth work requires an equally precise form of management.

## What is detached youth work?

It is not implicit that detached youth workers can 'deliver outcomes' on behalf of other services. Which is precisely the demand made of them by others who struggle to engage young people. This is to misunderstand how, and why, detached youth work works. It's precisely because detached youth workers don't start from a prescribed agenda that they are successful in meeting the needs of young people. Prescribing these outcomes hampers the very methodology that enables the work to be effective.

The Joseph Rowntree Foundation-commissioned national study of street-based youth work articulates this point well:

> This study suggests that when street-based work 'works', it does so because the young people who are the targets of interventions allow it to. In almost all the projects surveyed or visited, the work is based upon the voluntary participation of young people and the negotiation of roles and goals between them and the workers. It is also the case that low, medium and high need/risk young people often associate together and in many instances low-need/risk youngsters may provide a way into work with their higher need/risk peers. Moreover, most young people do not appear to be amenable to single-issue interventions and most workers do not attempt them for that reason. This suggests that dialogue, and a willingness to begin with the issues and questions that have significance for the young people, may well be a prerequisite for success, irrespective of whether street-based interventions have a primary concern with health, community safety, youth justice or education, training and employment.
>
> (Crimmens et al., 2004: 73)

The reality of detached youth work is that it is more and more targeted, more and more issue-based, and more and more 'programme-led' (Tiffany, 2007a: 50). One wonders whether policy makers, and indeed managers, are aware of this trend. Crimmens et al. offer a broader definition of detached youth work in response to this impoverished reality:

> Detached youth work endeavours to provide a broad-based, open-ended social education in which the interests, problems and issues to be dealt with, and the manner in which they are dealt with, emerge from a dialogue between the young person and the youth worker. The work usually takes place on the street or in other public or commercial leisure facilities. Detached youth workers may target individuals, groups, youth networks, adult networks or local administrative or political structures in an attempt to achieve beneficial change for young people.
>
> (Crimmens et al., 2004: 14)

Some central themes are worth highlighting. First, and perhaps most profoundly, this defines detached youth work as a form of education – a form of education that emphasises social learning through conversation and the experience of democracy (Jeffs and Smith, 1999: 119). That these conversations tend to take place in public space only adds to the inherent uncertainty of this kind of practice. But detached youth work, perhaps unusually, does not fear this. Rather it identifies these spaces as essential environments for learning.

> It is so important that teenagers are able to live elsewhere, in places where they can escape both family constraints and those of the systematic learning of rationale [school] ... in truth, it is this participation in social life within frameworks that are relatively free from the family and school sphere that guarantees the gradual emergence of autonomy in adolescence.
>
> (Meirieu, 1992: 1–5)

We now see more clearly one of the greatest challenges for managers of detached youth work: How should this uncertainty-based model be managed? Once again, clarity on rationale is what is needed, particularly as the current context of integrated services does not assume managers have knowledge of detached youth work. Put simply, detached youth work is designed to work with young people for whom uncertainty is a daily reality. Typically, behaviours and lifestyles are often chaotic and adherence to so-called norms less likely. It is simple enough to say that we need to work with this reality, but it is much harder to do. And, as a consequence, it is difficult to manage. Arnold et al. (1981) offer a spectrum that helps to clarify the young people detached youth workers work with (Figure 10.1).

In Figure 10.1 the indices X and Y represent a continuum of social exclusion/inclusion, along which different young people might be located. We can see that detached youth work seeks to engage those young people who, for a variety of often complex reasons, are not present in club and project work. Outreach work, we might note, also works toward the end of the spectrum that indicates social exclusion, but has the intention of taking a specific service out into the community; or 'reaching out' in order to bring young people back to a building-based provision. In sum, detached youth work is different because of its intention *not* to adopt a prescriptive stance, aware as it is that this can act as a barrier to the engagement of some young people, who seek much more tailored support.

But what does it take to work at this end of the spectrum? First, we have to be mindful of the complexity of why young people don't engage with these other structures. These range from simply not knowing the provision exists, to a fear that they would not be welcome in those places, or the fact that they may well have been banned from them before. The latter tends to represent a dissonance between the rules

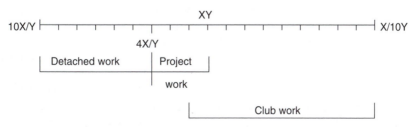

*Figure 10.1* A youth work spectrum (Arnold et al., 1981: 3)

these institutions insist upon, and those the young people are prepared to play by. Ultimately, young people may judge that they don't fit in and avoid these services as a consequence. Mainstream services therefore rarely have contact with them. Recognising this, the detached youth worker judges that the way to engage with young people is to meet them in the spaces they have confidence in and build the relationships through which help and support can be offered more successfully.

To engage young people in this way, certain principles need to be followed. First, there has to be a commitment 'to be as easily accessible as possible' (Dynamo International, 2009: 16), to work in a 'low threshold' manner (BAST, 2011). This entails being constantly aware of the things services do that constitute barriers to engagement. Some are real, some are perceived by young people; either way, they all prevent access. Low threshold practice is therefore about working to remove as many of these barriers as possible. It is about making services as accessible as possible; but not in the sense that we have to make it as easy as possible for young people to come to us. It is something more substantive and radical; it inverts the belief that *they* have to come to *us*. Typically, we might think about a building-based service with opening times that don't suit young people; where that building is in a place that is difficult to get to; where the 'gate-keepers' insist that the young person makes an appointment, and provides particular information (often sensitive) about themselves in advance. In each case, the threshold can be said to have been raised, such that the young person decides that it is not going to work for them.

Low threshold practice implies fluidity and creativity, being flexible, constantly negotiating boundaries, in order to be responsive to young people. Above all, it values proximity – getting close to young people; in essence, always trying to see the world from the young person's point of view. If this means that workers have to work in different places, at different times of the day, and work different hours from one week to the next, then this is the action that should be taken. It is the responsibility therefore of both detached youth workers and their managers to promote low threshold practice. Anything else simply reduces the capacity to engage and build relationships with young people who rarely, if ever, access services elsewhere. Thereafter, these relationships constitute the foundation on which young people can learn to access other services. You can't build on relationships that haven't been established.

Practically, detached youth workers listen out for and solicit a 'request' (Dynamo International, 2009: 42). These are the things young people ask workers to help them with. They are important for a number of reasons. First, they allow the workers to tap in to the things young people are interested in and intrinsically motivated by, fully aware that where young people lack motivation, this too, represents a barrier. Second, this implies, once again, being flexible and responsive. And it draws attention to the tensions implicit in prescribed, issue-based agendas; they risk being interpreted by young people as oppressive, or as someone seeking to coerce them. The consequence of all this is that the detached youth worker needs to know what is happening in the lives of young people, both generally and in their communities, and specifically in terms of their experiences, influences, trials, tribulations, hopes and fears. This is knowledge they cannot do without.

Forgive this wider context, but it was necessary in order to be able to argue that this has to be the starting point for the effective management of detached youth work; how can this knowledge be accessed by the worker; how can the manager help them to learn these things?

## The tensions and challenges of detached youth work management

Many of the tensions and challenges of managing in this context should now be apparent, but they are worth reiterating in our quest to identify an ideal type of management for detached youth work.

Misunderstanding of detached youth work is of particular concern. This is sometimes exacerbated by, but not exclusive to, the context of integrated services, where detached youth workers are frequently asked to work alongside other professionals in more formal ways (Davies and Merton, 2010). As a consequence, those managing detached youth work are increasingly unlikely to have knowledge or experience of detached youth work or even youth work backgrounds. Of course, many managers take it upon themselves to gain such knowledge and experience. But without this commitment it is all too common to see managers seduced by prescriptive outcomes-based models of practice, which are counter-productive in meeting the needs of those alienated from mainstream services (Tiffany, 2007b). This lack of understanding sees detached youth workers being set an increasing number of issue-based targets. They are forced into the very programme-led activities that are so unappealing to the very young people detached youth work has historically aimed to support.

In an attempt to fix this problem of its own making, policy increasingly impels workers to target individuals who have come to the attention of other services or who are identified through an increasingly spurious Risk Factor Prevention Paradigm (that mechanism by which we decide who precisely is 'at risk'), criticisms of which abound (Gray, 2005; Case, 2006; 2007; Goldson and Muncie, 2006; France, 2007; O'Mahoney, 2009).

This process of individuation represents no less than the de-socialisation of both detached youth work and wider youth work practice. Its roots are profoundly neo-liberal and managerialist, in that, it promotes the pathologisation of the individual and the degradation of any meaningful analysis of structural and political determinants to young people's problems. Worse still, a lack of awareness of detached youth work's socio-educational tradition sees it more and more directed at control-oriented strategies (de St Croix, 2010) and less and less 'youth-led' (Whelan, 2010: 57). The needs of the wider community often trump those of young people, as evidenced by the language of 'hot-spotting', 'rapid reaction' and 'community reassurance'. In sum, what is happening to detached youth work is indicative of a wider positivist approach to the management of public services (Haynes, 2003), in which there is a belief that an idealised type of management exists and this can then be universally applied.

If we are to address these concerns and support an account of detached youth which achieves good outcomes precisely because it is principled, certain management issues have to be tackled. In the first instance, the most obvious question to be addressed is: 'what underpins this interest in detached youth work, and do these interests relate substantively to the interests and concerns of young people?' What rationale informs this interest; and what kind of information do we judge as valuable in our decision-making? It seems obvious to say that we need some form of evidence that a need for detached youth work exists, and that detached youth work is a reasonable, appropriate and desirable response to this need. My aim in labouring a definition of detached youth work has been to support this judgement, by illustrating how important it is to be clear about what detached youth work is, and what the aims of detached youth work are. It is only then that we can reasonably validate the information needed to manage detached youth work effectively. The crux of the matter relates to a fundamental aspect of all management: *information*. Judging something to be informative and useful depends on what we take the concept of information to mean and our judgement about whether that material fits these criteria.

## 'Intelligence' based management

Despite its connotations with policing and espionage, thinking of information as intelligence (or not, as the case may be) offers a useful steer. It clarifies what information is actually important and what is useful in managerial decision-making. Let us say, simplistically, that intelligence is that material that makes us more intelligent. We can conclude, for detached youth work to meet the needs of young people, intelligence needs to flow primarily and substantively from the ground upwards, from the experiences and opinions of young people. It should not be dominated by the views of others.

The manager's principal task is therefore to access this intelligence. But what has our contextual analysis thus far shown? Working in this way is typically in direct contrast to a seemingly all-pervasive management model in which information is cascaded from on high. We see then that an alternative is called for; the model proposed actually inverts the dominant perspective. This has repercussions also for how we view managerial hierarchies and leaves us with another significant conclusion (as we also saw argued in Chapter 4): something more democratic is called for. Once again, our emerging model seems to reflect more and more the detached youth work process itself, and certainly the value base that underpins it.

Ignoring for a moment a much-needed critique of the neoliberal framing of young people as 'customers' of youth services, it is interesting to note that these democratic models are much in evidence in the theory of management:

> Decentralised – moving from hierarchy to participation and teams. Greater discretion for decision-making is pushed down the line to those staff who have direct contact with customers. The principle of subsidiarity is followed, i.e. decisions are made nearest to the ground unless they are better made higher up. Managers empower employees by flattening the chain of command and making sure that people are aware of what authority they have to act. Hand in hand with this empowerment, managers must establish clear processes for reporting back and accountability.
>
> (Ford et al., 2005: 112)

This is a central element of a new model of public sector management presented by Osbourne and Gaebler (1992). But – and it is a big 'but' – there is little evidence of this in detached youth work or, in youth work, or for that matter public services generally. The current climate is associated with:

> A rise of the managerialist culture – working with clear, explicit, processes to achieve measurable results against explicit targets. This contrasts with historic forms of professional management in which the professional was trained to a high level and then largely left to use his or her judgement in the delivery of services.

This can be characterised as a shift from 'Trust me (I am a professional)' to 'Prove it (and if you cannot I will sue)'.

(Ford et al., 2005: 110)

As we have seen at various points throughout this book, the management of youth work has been substantively reframed in this neoliberal context; and this is especially so in the case of detached youth work. The argument here is that *managers of detached youth work must reclaim progressive theories of management if the practice is to be successful in meeting the needs of the young people* it purports to help. So how do we achieve this? The value base of detached youth work has proved already to be useful in thinking about how it should be managed. But it is the practice of it that takes us even further. Detached youth work's emphasis on listening and talking to young people shows this is the way to achieving good outcomes. Might we say that management should adopt this 'communicative paradigm' also?

This is essential if we are to say that what we do is youth work *and* respond to the challenges of a context where the identification of need is increasingly externalised, i.e. detached youth work is more and more employed to meet others' needs, rather than those of young people.

This shift is evidence also of a growing disregard for genuine needs analysis, that process of 'reconnaissance' that provides the information on which decisions about the development of detached youth work projects were historically based (Goetchius and Tash, 1967; Arnold et al., 1981). In the main, this information was, and (it is argued) needs to be, accessed through conversations with the host community, and particularly with the young people who live there. Other research evidence, such as indices of deprivation, complement, rather than supplant, this. Reconnaissance then offers the possibility of a thorough analysis of what is actually happening on the ground, in that community. It aims to build an evidence base capable of illuminating the causes of the concerns that have been identified and the thinking behind a detached youth work response. Reconnaissance has the capacity to critically analyse perceptions, thereby objectifying social reality and helping to manage external expectations. It prompts a range of important questions:

Is the need identified verifiable (is it that of the young people)?
Is detached youth work the best way of meeting this need?
What is it that this vision of detached youth work hopes to achieve?
And, 'Do you have the flexibility/capacity to cope with the changes that detached work will bring?'

(Arnold et al., 1981: 16)

Ideally, a report based on the outcomes of this analysis is compiled. Such a document will hold weight in the often difficult discussions that need to take place with other agencies to secure agreement about why and how the project will work. Communicating these aims to the wider world becomes the next challenge. Many stakeholders might not have been integral to determining these aims, but they have a right to know and be clear about what is happening, and why. Having these aims written down in the form of a report helps clarify this and managers should therefore treat this as a priority. This is part of the wider managerial challenge of promoting and publicising detached youth work in order that it is understood by the widest audience. As we have seen, this is particularly important in the context of multi-agency working and integrated services.

### Supervision, faith and trust in detached youth work

Supervision should be an ongoing process. The detached youth worker is and continues to be the primary conduit of information to managers. Participatory research with young people complements this. Managers need to create a supportive culture amenable to these processes. Specifically, front-line workers need training and encouragement to be able to record, analyse and report on their learning from conversations with young people and the wider community. Supervision is the mechanism by which this happens. However, as we saw documented in Chapter 7, managerialism has restricted this practice to an almost exclusive focus upon accountability, to the detriment of its supportive and educative functions. Arguably detached youth workers are most in need of 'genuine' supervision, given the isolated nature of their work. Without it, intelligence gathering is compromised.

Thinking about supervision also helps in another respect. It reminds us once again that detached youth work values are applicable also to its management. Supervision, Kitto argues, has a core function of enabling reflections upon, and thinking critically about, practice (Kitto, 1993: 6). This aligns it with the autonomy and trust-enhancing interventions of good youth work. And it fits with the communicative and democratic paradigm of the work itself. Of particular note is how managing in this way helps workers identify not only what they can do, but also what they are not best suited to do. In low threshold practices this is essential, because our thinking must always focus on what works best for young people. This implies the value of a team work approach. Managers then have the added advantage of being able to distribute tasks, including deciding which workers are best placed to engage with which young people. Encouraging a strong team culture will mitigate any interpretation that this division of labour is a slight on individual capabilities. All become sympathetic to the simple reality that particular personal traits can act as an inhibitor to contact-making and engagement with those who are hardest to reach. Trying to work with a group of a particular ethnicity, for example, might necessitate the involvement of a role model from the same community. Where there's a strong collaborative culture, premised on working in the best interests of young people, workers will be more prepared to pass the baton to a colleague, as appropriate.

### Conclusion

The argument presented is relatively straightforward: the outcomes so many stakeholders hope for depend on a sound theoretical understanding of what detached youth work is, how it works and the values that underpin it, followed by practical work based solidly on that understanding. It is of great concern that an analysis of the current context affecting detached youth work reveals otherwise. This represents the greatest challenge for detached workers and their managers. But recognising the managerialist roots of this problem points the finger squarely at managers; and begs the fundamental question: are they part of the problem or part of the solution?

It might be a step too far to conclude that detached youth work needs minimal or even no management, a return perhaps to the early days of youth work management, as outlined by Davies in Chapter 1, where the manager fulfils no more than an advisory role. Nonetheless, it is arguable that detached youth workers would achieve much more with minimal managerial interference, especially that influenced by neoliberal and managerialist perspectives, that only seems to constrain their practice. It is certainly true that an increasing array of demands and drivers impact on detached youth work and that these need to be managed, and managed strongly. Many more voices want a say in what detached youth workers do, and where they do it. The effective management of these external relationships is essential if detached youth workers are to be supported in low threshold practices, dependent as they are on flexibility, accessibility and professional judgement in pursuit of 'what works'. This has to be a managerial priority. So too is support for workers as the primary conduit through which that vital intelligence, so fundamental to achieving good outcomes, flows – primarily from young people, through detached workers, to management; and not the other way round.

## Questions for reflection and discussion

1  What are the constituents of 'low threshold' practice, and how do detached youth workers maximise the engagement of young people?
2  What is the basis of 'intelligence based management', how is information gathered, and how is the upward flow of this information ensured?
3  What is the future of detached youth work? How can this distinct form of practice best be supported, and managed?

## Further reading

Crimmens, D., Factor, F., Jeffs, T., Pitts, J., Pugh, C., Spence, J. and Turner, P. (2004) *Reaching Socially Excluded Young People: A National Study of Street-based Youth Work*, Leicester: Joseph Rowntree Foundation.
Tiffany, G. A. (2007a) *Reconnecting Detached Youth Work: Guidelines and Standards for Excellence*, Leicester: Federation for Detached Youth Work.
Whelan, M. (2010) 'Detached youth work', in Batsleer, J. and Davies, B. (eds) *What Is Youth Work?* Exeter: Learning Matters, 47–60.

## References

Arnold, J., Askins, D., Davies, R., Evans, S., Rogers, A. and Taylor, T. (1981) *The Management of Detached Youth Work: How and Why*, Leicester: Youth Clubs UK (now UK Youth: www.ukyouth.org).
BAST (2011) (Bundesarbeitsgemeinschaft Straßensozialarbeit Österreich (Austrian Working Committee of Social Streetwork) www.bast.at/en/streetwork/ (Accessed 10/01/2011).
Case, S. (2006) 'Young people "at risk" of what? Challenging risk-focused early intervention as crime prevention', *Youth Justice*, 6(3): 171–79.
——(2007) 'Questioning the evidence of risk that underpins evidence-led youth justice intervention', *Youth Justice*, 7(2): 91–105.
CNLAPS (2008) (Comité National de Liaison des Associations de Prevéntion Spécialisée), Seminaire International de Formation sur le Travail de Rue dans le Monde, 27–28 November, La Ciotat, France.
Crimmens, D., Factor, F., Jeffs, T., Pitts, J., Pugh, C., Spence, J. and Turner, P. (2004) *Reaching Socially Excluded Young People: A National Study of Street-based Youth Work*, Leicester: Joseph Rowntree Foundation.
de St Croix, T. (2010) 'Youth work and the surveillance state', in Batsleer, J. and Davies, B. (eds) *What Is Youth Work?* Exeter: Learning Matters, pp. 140–52.
Davies, B. and Merton, B. (2010) 'Straws in the wind: the state of youth work practice in a changing policy environment', *Youth and Policy*, Winter, no. 105: 9–36.

Dynamo International (The International Network of Social Street workers) (2009) *International Guide on the Methodology of Street Work Throughout the World*, Brussels: Dynamo International.

Ford, K., Hunter, R., Merton, B. and Waller, D. (2005) *Leading and Managing Youth Work and Services for Young People*, Leicester: National Youth Agency.

France, A. (2007) 'Risk factor analysis and the youth question', *Journal of Youth Studies*, 11(1): 1–15.

Goetchius, G. and Tash, M. J. (1967) *Working with Unattached Youth: Problem, Approach, Method*, London: Routledge and Kegan Paul.

Goldson, B. and Muncie, J. (2006) 'Rethinking youth justice: comparative analysis, international human rights and research evidence', *Youth Justice*, 6(2): 91–106.

Gray, P. (2005) 'The politics of risk and young offenders' experiences of social exclusion and restorative justice', *British Journal of Criminology*, 45: 938–57.

Haynes, P. (2003) *Managing Complexity in the Public Services*, Berkshire: Open University Press.

Jeffs, T. and Smith, M. K. (1999) *Informal Education: Conversation, Democracy and Learning*, Ticknall, Derbyshire: Education Now.

Kitto, J. (1986) *Holding the Boundaries: Professional Training of Face to Face Workers at a Distance*, London: YMCA National College.

——(1993) 'The Nature of Supervision', in *Developing Professional Practice*, study pack CFS301, Unit 1, Certificate in Supervision. London: YMCA George Williams College.

Meirieu, P. (1992) 'Mais comment peut-on être adolescent?', Belgian Street Workers' Workshop, Brussels, 21 October, pp. 1–5. Also in *Pédagogie collègiale*, 6(2): 29–32.

O'Mahoney, P. (2009) 'The risk factors prevention paradigm and the causes of youth crime: a deceptively useful analysis?', *Youth Justice*, 9(2), available at www.iprt.ie/files/Dr_Paul_O_Mahony_Journal_Article_in_Youth_Justice_Riskproof.pdf (accessed 11/01/2011).

Osbourne, D. and Gaebler, T. (1992) *Reinventing Government: How the Entrepreneurial Spirit Is Transforming the Public Sector*, Boston, MA: Addison-Wesley.

Smith, M. K. (2007) 'Classic studies in informal education: working with unattached youth', *The Encyclopaedia of Informal Education*, www.infed.org/research/working_with_unattached_youth.htm (accessed 07/04/2011).

Tiffany, G. A. (2007a) *Reconnecting Detached Youth Work: Guidelines and Standards for Excellence*, Leicester: Federation for Detached Youth Work.

——(2007b) 'Lessons from the street: informal education-based social ties building and the danger of pre-scription', in *Ville, lien social, intervention sociale*, Brussels: Pensée plurielle, no. 15–2007/2, De Boeck Université. www.cairn.info/load_pdf.php?ID_ARTICLE=PP_015_0129

Whelan, M. (2010) 'Detached youth work', in Batsleer, J. and Davies, B. (eds) *What Is Youth Work?* Exeter: Learning Matters, pp. 47–60.

# Part III

# The settings of youth work management

# 11 Managing youth work in integrated services

*Bernard Davies and Bryan Merton*

This chapter attempts to both describe, and analyse, youth work management in the current context of integrated services. It draws on some recent research carried out for De Montfort University (DMU) by the authors (Davies and Merton, 2009a; 2009b; 2010; Davies 2010) as well as lessons learnt from a series of leadership and management development programmes for the youth sector, commissioned by the Children's Workforce Development Council, delivered by Ford Management Partnership. This included the Leadership Enhancement Programme (LEP) and the Leadership Development Programme (LDP) 2009–10. Together these programmes reached over 500 strategic and aspiring leaders in both the local authority and voluntary and community sectors working in the context of integrated services. This chapter does not claim to be definitive but attempts to offer some preliminary findings to 'shed a light upon' a complex, uncertain and ever changing managerial situation, which existed before the major cuts in public spending were implemented in 2010 and beyond.

## Policy framework of integrated services

Informal and ad hoc partnership arrangements have arguably existed for many years within youth work, both between statutory and voluntary services as well as between youth work agencies and other related professions (Harrison et al., 2003). However, a step change in partnership and integrated working arrived with the election of the first New Labour government in 1997. As we saw in Chapter 2, 'joined up government' and 'partnership working' were a high priority for New Labour. The early attempts to promote and encourage 'joined up' working were introduced under the auspices of Connexions (DfES, 2000), described as 'The best start in life for every young person' (DfES, 2001b). Connexions was an initial attempt to integrate support services for all young people aged 13–19. Early plans included suggestions that the youth service would be wholly absorbed into the new service outside local authority control, generating some persisting tensions.

> '[While] we have to do all the hard graft and help get the young people ready for EET opportunities ... they [Connexions] take the credit for the placement'.
>
> (Davies and Merton, 2010: 32)

With a priority focus on the socially excluded, it emphasized personal advice, support and guidance and created a new role of 'personal adviser'. The service was both 'universal' (open to everyone) but also 'targeted' (catering for the most in need).

Connexions was also described as both a service and strategy, and this often created confusion about which aspect youth work related to. As we shall see, this lack of clarity often continued into the creation of integrated services.

Arguably, Connexions had not resulted in the breakdown of what Margaret Hodge MP was later to refer to as the 'silo' mentality (Hodge, 2005: 2). The desired changes in integration that government policy-makers had required were finally brought about by Every Child Matters (ECM, DfES, 2003), and later Youth Matters (DfES, 2005; 2006), which followed the 'politicization' of the tragic death of Victoria Climbié. This encouraged greater integration of the previously discrete and arguably disparate services for young people such as social services, education and criminal justice (though this time within local authority structures rather than the Connexions Partnerships). No longer were youth services permitted to be merely part of an overall integrated 'strategy'. They were to be restructured within Children's Trusts, and become part of a brave new world of integrated service delivery.

Integrating youth work into the new children and young people's structures did not of course take place in a policy vacuum. Indeed, the DMU research revealed that managers and field workers were only too aware of a range of New Labour policy priorities which often were driven by the same broad objectives as the integration agenda (DfES, 2002; 2005; 2006; DCSF, 2007c). Perhaps most notable of these was enabling young people to achieve accredited and recorded outcomes (DfES, 2002; Flint, 2005), and strengthening their 'voice and influence' within decision-making processes. In addition expectations were placed on youth work services to target young people identified as 'at risk' or 'risky'; i.e. 'NEETs', actual or potential offenders, teenage parents, drug abusers (DfCSF, 2007b). Even ostensibly more open-ended policies – for example increasing young people's participation in 'positive activities' and extending weekend evening facilities – had the often explicit goal of tackling 'anti-social behaviour' by creating diversionary provision (DfCSF, 2007a; Hillier, 2009).

One consequence of these targeting pressures was to draw youth work managers more directly and more deeply into 'partnership working' with other agencies outside their traditional education locations, such as health, police, or youth offending teams (YOTs). Notwithstanding the benefits this could bring, some managers suggested this provided challenges for youth work:

> a lot of what we do is linked in to key partners – parish council, police, Youth Offending Team. We make (those links) by revisiting core principles because partners have to be clear and we have to be clear what we are bringing.
>
> (Senior manager, in Davies and Merton, 2009a: 34)

## Uncertainty of integration

Change is a constant in all modern public services (Ford et al., 2005; Tyler et al., 2009) and integrated youth services is no different. However it would appear that not only has the complexity increased but it has involved a much more concerted effort to achieving integration than previous policy emphasis on 'partnership'. Still in its infancy, integrated services were subject to a great deal of turbulence where organizational maps and service plans were being reviewed and redrawn. New teams of professional workers were brought together to work with young people and their families. Staff had to adjust to new priorities and ways of working with colleagues from different professional disciplines. Funding streams were introduced, then reduced and in some cases[1] later disappeared altogether. Officers operated along different lines of management, reporting and accountability, sometimes including so-called 'matrix' arrangements[2] combining a series of processes that were complex and time-consuming. Staff were deployed in different formations, often in localities, where youth workers worked alongside other professionals such as Connexions, education welfare and social services and had little if any contact with other youth workers. Furthermore, some may have been line managed by someone without specific youth work knowledge or skills. Planning and decision-making were increasingly provisional and short-term. All this created a pervasive climate of uncertainty and unease that made management *exceptionally demanding*.

Participants in the two leadership and development programmes shared their uncertainty about the locus of control and the sphere of influence in their work. For many this produced considerable anxiety because they were not clear about what they were responsible for and what criteria they were being judged by. If they themselves were not clear, then those they managed were likely to be even less clear. Managers of integrated youth support on the LEP and LDP were judged to excel in understanding, working with, and on behalf, of young people. Unsurprisingly the aspect of leadership that managers were consistently weaker at was clarifying expectations for those whom they managed, and giving their staff clear and consistent feedback about how they were performing. It was no surprise therefore that the managers' unease was passed down the line, generating feelings of disempowerment.

A concern was expressed by some service managers that government had deliberately not provided a blueprint, leaving it to local interests to create their own means of planning and delivering integrated youth support service; as one worker suggested: 'no one has defined it'. This meant much time was spent looking inwards at structures and processes within the local authority rather than outwards at developing a broader vision of working together with new partners. This exacerbated the uncertainty, with many managers admitting that they themselves were not yet clear about the local interpretation of the policy for integrated youth support. 'It's been 18 months and I still don't know what my job is … now no-one knows' (senior manager, in Davies and Merton, 2009a: 39). As a result there was confusion about what exactly was being integrated in the youth support sector. Did integration refer to services, structure or strategy, or was it any permutation of all three?

### Services and structures

Once the implementation of children's trusts, the formal structures enabling integration of services within the local authorities, began to take shape, a key question for youth work was which other services it would be structurally linked with. The youth service and Connexions provided a useful starting point. Those that included youth offending did meet some resistance, since much of its funding and policy direction came from the Youth Justice Board, an entirely different source. There was some confusion too about the types of service to be integrated; were they to be the universal services (notionally available to all but actually rationed to some), targeted services aimed at those at risk or disadvantaged, or specialist services directed towards those who have particular needs, conditions or interests?

However, this was not always easy to discern, and large variations existed across the country. One youth work manager was clear that her authority had gone for 'evolution rather than revolution' – 'a salad rather than a soup' approach which was informally managed. Here as in one or two other authorities, even within the changed structures, versions of integration seemed to be operating which remained heavily reliant on individual managers' and indeed workers' flair and initiative. Power and politics would inevitably come into play. In one large authority which promoted the principal youth officer to the position of head of integrated youth support services (IYSS) the youth service remaining largely intact and a senior manager described the situation as: 'we continue to promote and celebrate the partnership work we have always done, it's really just virtual integration'. In such cases, as we shall see below, integration became something of a mystery for many of the field staff. However, in many other situations where youth work managers were less influential new structures emerged which brought together disparate groupings of professionals, sometimes in co-located teams. The divisions or directorates which emerged had titles which included 'targeted services' (for example encompassing youth offending), 'fostering, residential care and adoption', 'access to education' (including SEN and 'inclusion'), 'prevention and safeguarding', 'vulnerable children' and 'access, inclusion and participation'.

Examples of the structural changes to youth work and their 'new' location included:

- A youth service located within a community services directorate which also had responsibility for youth offending; children and families, early intervention, voice and influence, and disability and parenting services.
- Universal provision and positive activities with a lead officer with responsibility also for the voluntary and community sector, equalities, participation and young people's volunteering and safeguarding.
- A young people's service located in a directorate for safeguarding and specialist services whose overall responsibilities included child protection, child care and child disability, family support, preventative services and youth offending. The young people's service itself incorporated family support services for children and young people over 11, for children who were looked after and leaving care and for fostering and adoption, and included a post of youth work manager.
- Integrated and targeted support for young people located in a directorate of targeted and early intervention services which, through a young people's service, provided locality-commissioned support for young people, targeted youth support, and information, advice and guidance.

The reasons for the particular grouping of services were not always apparent. Indeed, reflecting on her own local authority's decisions, one middle manager concluded:

> Strategically it's a weird arranged marriage – I won't say forced! … Why put together *those* services [youth offending service; Connexions]? Why not youth work with the schools and colleges? The reasons for the links aren't clear … Workers … may be far closer to other people [services outside IYSS than those located within it].
>
> (Davies and Merton, 2010: 30)

## Effects of integration

Although it often remained unclear precisely how integration was to be implemented, youth work managers were already dealing with some significant challenges. As one manager suggested, the demands of partnership working had already undermined some of the managerial functions:

> We've moved from managing staff and projects to managing partnerships ... the demands of joining up have eroded some of our quality assurance processes – no longer visiting centres (for practice observation) as we once did.
>
> (Davies and Merton, 2009a: 40)

The LEP and LDP research found that some senior youth work managers talked of high levels of interference from – indeed of micro-management by – their departmental senior managers. In addition the lengthening internal hierarchies and changing departmental priorities, were for some senior youth work managers starting to be experienced as personally, as well as professionally, oppressive: 'It's now just hard. I've never worked as hard – as long hours' (Davies and Merton, 2010: 54).

## *Complexity*

One of the primary effects of integrated services communicated by managers was the increased complexity. 'A massive range [of tasks] ... Translating strategy into practice' (Davies and Merton, 2010: 54). For example, managers had to deal with competing demands on time and attention from different quarters requiring relentless prioritizing and decision-making, sometimes with incomplete information and inadequate analysis. Managers were expected to respond to pressures from myriad competing and some-times conflicting stakeholders with their respective agendas and at the same time come up with new ideas, plans and programmes. Evidence from the LDP and LEP showed that managers were required to be both strategic and to attend to operational matters such as budget setting, asset maintenance, staff deployment, performance management, and risk assessments. They had to make connections between policies, programmes and provision and draw up plans and interventions which simultaneously addressed their inter-relationship. They had to deal with some problems that had precedents and lend themselves to multiple solutions (and choose one) and others that lent themselves to none that were immediately apparent. They may have had access to specialist expertise and resources or they may not. They were instructed to transform at the same time as maintain continuity and stability.

It is clear from the LEP and LDP that few managers have been sufficiently trained to handle the resulting complexity. For example, they have had little encouragement to create environments and experiments that allow for solutions to emerge, and then seek and make sense of advice on how to proceed that may be different and sometimes conflicting; or to engage in open thinking that invites multiple scenarios. Managers reported difficulty in moving beyond accepted methods of problem solving, and found it hard to engage in a process of waiting, watching, analysing and then intervening; as well as to differentiate between simple, complex and chaotic contexts and situations and then judge responses best suited to each. Managers could not be expected to inherently possess the intellectual rigour and emotional resilience required for mana-ging such complexity. These were qualities that could be developed. The key question was whether there existed sufficient commitment to invest in professional development opportunities that gave leaders and managers the time and mental space to acquire the models, skills, tools and techniques that would assist them in this difficult process.

It should be remembered that partnerships are not formed overnight (Moss Kanter, 1994; Harrison et al., 2003). They require patient and careful nurturing, as people from different agencies and professional backgrounds develop an understanding of each other and seek to create the conditions of trust and mutual regard that are vital if the new integrated arrangements are to work well. Similarly this process requires both time and investment in staff development, a 'luxury' not always afforded to the newly formed children's trusts. Of equal importance are the channels of communication established within the new patterns of integrated services, requiring an emphasis on both lateral and upwards communication (Cole, 2004) as well as on the traditional view of managerial communication as cascading downwards from the top of the hierarchy.

Perhaps surprisingly nonetheless, many, perhaps even most, of the managers interviewed remained positive about the 'principle' of integration: 'I'm over the moon we've got an integrated service, especially for young people with multiple issues' (head of IYSS, in Davies and Merton, 2010: 28). Many too, were optimistic about its actual operation. One senior manager talked of a management team (of which they were a member) which now included all services, a single referral route into the CAF process and a strategy paper aiming in the future for 'inter-disciplinary location' (Davies and Merton, 2010: 29). A middle manager in another service commented: 'Those walls are down now. I like it: it stops people staying in their own environment' (Davies and Merton, 2009a: 35). Some workers too were supportive of what was happening: 'I have been keen to integrate services for years' (Davies and Merton, 2010: 31).

### Gap between managers and practitioners

However, there often seemed to be a marked gap in both the experience, and perception, of integration separating managers and their workers, which if anything was widening. As we have seen, managers reported that they had less time for visiting clubs and supporting workers. As one middle management team acknowledged, they were 'treading water', something which workers in another authority made explicit: 'Today is the first time I've seen (head of service) for months [and] when they do come it's usually bad news' (Davies and Merton, 2010: 51–52).

Even where there was good will – 'it [integration] could work here if it was done properly' – the message from below was at times riddled with confusion, asserting for example that integration was just not happening 'in practice'. Some workers suggested that 'We're not sharing practice' (Davies and Merton, 2010: 32) and that youth work was 'still a miniature professional island' with an 'appearance' of integration seen by field staff as 'all happening above us – just the senior people meeting' (Davies and Merton, 2010: 52). Even where managers talked of integration as a fact, their field staff were saying: 'I don't think it's been adopted here as much as elsewhere'. One worker even suggested that integrated services was merely: 'just a change of title – there have been no physical changes' (Davies and Merton, 2010: 31). While perhaps the most damning of all was the reaction of one group of ten full-time youth workers who greeted the mere mention of the word integration with uproarious, apparently cynical, laughter: 'It's nonsense … they make it up – to look good'.

Even where workers noticed a semblance of 'integrated working' they commented that there was a tendency to 'refer people to other agencies who work with them for six weeks. It's like passing the buck and nothing gets done' (Davies and Merton, 2010: 17). Some even suggested that the sharing of responsibility and joined up working had lessened as a result of more formal integrated structures, commenting that: 'The Connexions worker used to come to the youth centre. Now I have to ask them to come. There's never any feedback from the Connexions worker.'

### Implications for practice

One of the questions facing youth work with its 'relocation' into integrated services, whether virtual or otherwise, was: Would its distinctive form of practice survive, and thrive? Within these new arrangements youth work was embroiled in differing, but often crucial, political and power relationships, with varied results. In one (small) authority, the head of IYSS was sufficiently identified with youth work to, very comfortably for all it seemed, take a full part in the group discussion. In another (middle size) authority, the youth work managers were clear that, albeit after a struggle, 'we've kept the youth work ethos by winning the argument [with senior departmental managers]' (Davies and Merton, 2010: 29). But by contrast, in another (much bigger) authority, though these did not seem to be consensus views, one senior manager commented that in the old education department: 'we had a place ... now there's no main heading', while another admitted: 'I'm not completely confident they [the department's senior management team] know our business' (Davies and Merton, 2010: 30).

On the LEP and LDP, concerns were expressed that youth work's connection with more developmental forms of education were being significantly weakened. One of the immediate concerns was that integrated services had reinforced the targeting of practice on 'at risk' and 'risky' young people and so emphasized the deficit model of young people. A second implication was to prioritize safeguarding agendas, which emphasized the paternalistic, welfare concerns of professionals rather than emphasized young people's right to self-determination and independence, focusing on their potential for development.

The effects on practice were perhaps most apparent in relation to protocols for recording and sharing young people's personal information, on whose actual implementation managers often had influence but which their field workers might resent, to such an extent that on occasion they would try to bypass or subvert them: 'I'm actively encouraging young people to go against the system. I say here's a form; please don't sign it ... I say [to my manager]: The young person says I can't share that' (Youth worker, in Davies and Merton, 2009a: 20). After pointing to often imaginative 'pockets of resistance' amongst young people themselves, De St Croix (2008; 2010) suggests that, as well as 'covert forms of opposition [which] are almost impossible to gauge', more overt resistance to these procedures also existed: 'I have fought my authority, I have fought and I fight ... to say I don't agree with this. I don't think we should be doing it' (De St Croix, 2010: 150–51).

However, a number of workers as well as managers were very positive about the benefits for young people of integration – such as the easier access it provided to other services and professionals. One manager reported, for example, 'I've just done the "Team Around the Child" training; I felt a real part of the group. ... youth work fitted in really well to the role play we did' (Davies and Merton, 2009: 36). Another concluded that: 'All the agencies know what everyone is doing' (Davies and Merton, 2010: 29). While a youth worker commented: 'The tone's changed. We are listened to, invited in – people want youth work as we define it' (Davies and Merton, 2009: 44).

Nonetheless, one experienced detached worker posed the question: whose interest ultimately is such joined up working serving?

On E2E there was a young person who a housing association was making homeless (for £200) ... I rang the office and said maybe we should pay the £200. I was told this was unprofessional ... I question whether our responsibility is to the housing association or to the young person. Management maybe have lost the way on that sort of thing.

(Davies and Merton, 2009: 34)

Despite the pressures on agencies and organizations within formal integrated services, partnerships with services 'outside' the new IYSS structures still appeared to be given considerable importance. This often increased the pressure on youth work and youth work management. For example, in one authority, area-based 'learning teams' were being developed chaired by a youth work manager and comprising youth workers, police, YOT and drugs workers. Close working relationships with the police emerged as a growing priority – for example, in the name of early intervention, 'triage' work in police stations was introduced in one authority 'to support young people in stressful situations'. Clearly requiring at times testing inter-agency cooperation, one senior youth work manager, commenting on the relationships required, reported that: 'We can have a "*close*" dialogue about what's *not* working well – tell the police managers and they'll listen' (Davies and Merton, 2010: 37–38).

## Commissioning

In line with the neoliberal ethos underpinning New Labour's policy initiatives, an explicit challenge for children's trusts was to develop the commissioning process for youth work delivery in order to ensure competition (DfES, 2005; 2006; DfCSF, 2007a). Whilst some services interpreted this in a limited capacity, for example in relation to the delivery and funding of positive activities, others saw it as an opportunity to 'contract out' a wider range of services. However, as we saw previously in Chapter 2, this is arguably not necessarily done in order to achieve higher quality of service but to do more for less. It was perhaps in the commissioning process that managerialism was most evident within the development of integrated services. Despite assurances that it was concerned with 'ensuring quality', the principle of the three E's of efficiency, effectiveness and economy (Farnham and Horton, 1993) were writ large. As one manager suggested: 'They keep asking for just a little bit more' (Davies and Merton, 2010: 54).

The LEP and LDP attempted to forge stronger relationships between the voluntary and community sector and the partners they had traditionally worked with in the local authority in providing services for young people. However, this did not always happen without a fair degree of mutual suspicion of the 'voluntary and community sector' expressing some uncertainty about their role and the expectations the statutory sector had of them. Communicating a vulnerability derived from their own limited capacity to influence, they also often complained of poor information and weak lines of communication. There was often too a lack of clarity about representation: who was to speak for the third sector when views were being canvassed and discussions about policies, priorities and procedures were being held?

Arrangements for commissioning services varied considerably from area to area. In some places local authorities were at the starting-gate, others were more advanced. At no matter what stage, however, the commissioning process exemplified the paradoxical status of 'partners' within children's trusts. As we saw earlier in Chapter 2, this simultaneously drew youth service providers into both cooperative and competitive relationships. Thus voluntary organizations could find themselves at the end of the pro-curement line without having any opportunity to contribute their experience and knowl-edge to the whole commissioning process (Davies and Merton, 2010: 33, 40). (For a more detailed analysis of the challenges of managing in the voluntary sector, see Chapter 13.)

## Conclusion

The available evidence suggests that marked differences existed in attitudes towards, and perceptions of, integrated services. Variations existed both between, as well as within, localities. In addition differences were also apparent between the attitudes of managers, who were often more committed and spoke positively about integrated services, and those of face-to-face workers who in general appeared more sceptical.

What was apparent too, however, was that the moves to integrated services had brought an unprecedented level of complexity into the management of youth work. It had also produced considerable difficulties for managers who found themselves having to balance competing demands and shifting expectations. A tension was evident between managers' commitment to ensuring the continuation of youth work as they defined it, and the need to make (sometimes substantial) concessions in order to accommodate the expectations and requirements of integrated services. The priorities of safeguarding young people but especially children, as well as combating 'anti-social beha-viour' were very high on the agenda of the emerging children's trusts and this impacted, often significantly, upon youth work priorities. Following the new Conservative/Liberal Democrat coalition's comprehensive spending review and the resulting 'major cuts' imposed on local authority spending, some of the trends identified in this research appeared to have become even more pronounced. The process was also exacerbated by the fall-out from the Baby Peter case in Haringey which concentrated service manager's minds even more sharply on 'safeguarding', and the avoidance of media scandals. Though much of the evidence remained at the level of reportage, a number of autho-rities announced their intention to in effect cease or substantially reduce funding what historically had been the core, even defining, form of youth work – open access provi-sion, attended by choice by young people, mainly in the form of the local youth club or centre (Hillier, 2010; Lepper, 2011). In Oxfordshire, for example, the council was pro-posing to close 20 of its 27 youth centres (Mahadevan, 2011), while Warwickshire indicated that it could 'cease the Youth Service' within four years (BBC, 2010). Where authorities did not then actually make youth workers redundant, they often planned to convert them into 'early intervention' workers with a largely social care role targeted at identified 'at risk' young people (see for example Lepper, 2010a; 2010b).

Doubtless the pace of change, originally initiated by the integration agenda, was further increasing as a result of the spending cuts. Those more likely to survive would, it appeared, be the targeted rather than the universal services, and geared much more specifically to the control of young people. For youth work managers within integrated services the dilemmas identified above thus seemed likely only to intensify.

## Questions for reflection and discussion

1   Reflect on youth work before integrated youth support services (IYSS) were estab-lished; what were the positives and negatives of 'partnership working' and your professional relationships with other services and agencies at that time? What are

the lessons for IYSS? (If you do not have experience of youth work prior to IYSS, talk to someone who has, about their experience.)

2   In your experience, in what ways has the integration of children and young people's services affected how youth work is *managed*? Identify and discuss any gains and losses in these developments.

3   In your experience, in what ways has the integration of children and young people's services affected the *practice* of youth work? Identify and discuss any gains and losses in these developments.

## Notes

1 Youth Capital Fund (YCF) and Youth Opportunities Fund (YOF) (Youth Matters, DfES, 2005; 2006), and Positive Activities for Young People (PAYP) (Aiming High, DfCSF, 2007a).

2 'Matrix management' involves a situation where an employee simultaneously has two managers: a 'functional manager' and a 'line manager'. Matrix management is a formal development of what is accepted as an inevitable consequence of the informal process of employees establishing links and networks across formal line management structures. Matrix management does have legitimacy in private sector management practices. As Hannagan (2008) describes: 'matrix structures usually involve managers being responsible to more than one senior manager, so that for one part of their work they will be line managed by one manager and for another part another ... usually based on a division between a functional management role and a project role' (Hannagan, 2008: 19). The idea is that the matrix enables an organization to maximize both 'vertical' and 'horizontal' communication and cooperation. This is, however, not without its problems. For youth work in integrated services this often means youth workers have a youth work manager who deals with professional issues and a locality manager (who is not a youth worker) who deals with line management issues; although inevitably questions about who deals with what, and who has ultimate responsibility, are likely to lead to confusion.

## Further reading

Batsleer, J. (2010) 'Youth work prospects: back to the future', in Davies, B. and Batsleer, J. (eds) *What Is Youth Work?* Exeter: Learning Matters, pp. 153–65.

Davies, B. and Merton, B. (2009) *Squaring the Circle? Findings of a 'Modest Inquiry' into the State of Youth Work Practice in a Changing Policy Environment*, Leicester De Montfort University, available at www.dmu.ac.uk/Images/Squaring%20the%20Circle_tcm6-50166.pdf

——(2010) *Straws in the Wind: The State of Youth Work Practice in a Changing Policy Environment (Phase 2)*, Leicester De Montfort University, available at www.dmu.ac.uk/Images/Straws%20in%20the%20Wind%20-%20Final%20Report%20-%20October%202010_tcm6-67206.pdf

Davies, B. and Wood, E. (2010) 'Youth work practice in integrated youth support services', in Davies, B. and Batsleer, J. (eds) *What Is Youth Work?* Exeter: Learning Matters, pp. 73–89.

Tyler, M., Hoggarth, L. and Merton, B. (2009) *Managing Modern Youth Work*, Exeter: Learning Matters, pp. 116–42.

## References

BBC (2010) 'Warwickshire County Council may cut youth services', www.bbc.co.uk/news/uk-england-coventry-warwickshire-11694304, 4 November, accessed 25 January 2011.

Cole, G. A. (2004) *Management Theory and Practice*, London: Thomson.

Davies, B. (2010) 'Straws in the wind: the state of youth work practice in a changing policy environment', *Youth and Policy*, Winter, no. 105: 9–36.

Davies, B. and Merton, B. (2009a) *Squaring the Circle?: Findings of a 'Modest Inquiry' into the State of Youth Work Practice in a Changing Policy Environment*, Leicester De Montfort University, available at www.dmu.ac.uk/Images/Squaring%20the%20Circle_tcm6-50166.pdf

——(2009b) 'Squaring the circle? The state of youth work in some children and young people's services', *Youth and Policy*, Summer, no. 103: 5–24.

——(2010) *Straws in the Wind: The State of Youth Work Practice in a Changing Policy Environment (Phase 2)*, Leicester De Montfort University, available at www.dmu.ac.uk/Images/Straws%20in%20the%20Wind%20-%20Final%20Report%20-%20October%202010_tcm6-67206.pdf

DCSF (2007c) 'Cash to provide positive activities for young people', available at www.dcsf.gov.uk/pns/DisplayPN.cgi?pn_id=2007_0231 (accessed 5 August 2010).

De St Croix, T. (2008) 'Swimming against the tide', detached.youthworkonline.org.uk/forum/topics/informal-education-or

——(2010) 'Youth work and the surveillance state', in Davies, B. and Batsleer, J. (eds) *What Is Youth Work?* Exeter: Learning Matters, pp. 140–52.

DfCSF (2007a) *Aiming High for Young People: A Ten Year Strategy for Positive Activities*, London: HMSO.

——(2007b) *Targeted Youth Support: A Guide*, London: HMSO.

DfES (2000) *Connexions: The Best Start in Life for Every Young Person*, www.lga.gov.uk/lga/parliament/connexions.pdf

——(2001) *Transforming Youth Work: Developing Youth Work for Young People*, London: HMSO.

——(2001b) *Understanding Connexions*, London: HMSO.

——(2002) *Transforming Youth Work: Resourcing Excellent Youth Services*, London: HMSO.

——(2003) *Every Child Matters*, London: HMSO.

——(2005) *Youth Matters*, London: HMSO.

——(2006) *Youth Matters: The Next Steps*, London: HMSO.

Farnham, D. and Horton, S. (eds) (1993) *Managing the New Public Services* (2nd edn 1996) Basingstoke: Macmillan.

Flint, W. (2005) *Recording Young People's Progress and Accreditation in Youth Work*, Leicester: NYA.

Ford, K., Hunter, R., Merton, B. and Waller, D. (2005) *Leading and Managing Youth Work and Services for Young People*, Leicester: NYA.

Hannagan, T. (2008) *Management Concepts and Practices* (5th edn) Harlow: Prentice Hall/Financial Times.

Harrison, R., Mann, G., Murphy, M., Taylor, A. and Thompson, N. (2003) *Partnership Made Painless: A Joined-up Guide to Working Together*, Lyme Regis: RHP.

Hillier, A. (2009), 'Hughes calls for more weekend youth activities', *Children and Young People Now*, 30 April. www.cypnow.co.uk

——(2010) 'True scale of youth service cuts around the corner', *Children and Young People Now*, 12 October. www.cypnow.co.uk

Hodge, M. (2005) 'The youth of today', Speech to Institute of Public Policy Research, 19 January.

Lepper, J. (2010a) 'West Sussex youth services hit by £2m cuts', *Children and Young People Now*, 4 August. www.cypnow.co.uk

——(2010b) 'Suffolk youth clubs under threat as council looks to a more targeted youth service', *Children and Young People Now*, 12 November. www.cypnow.co.uk

——(2011) 'Young people protest against cuts to Rotherham youth services', *Children and Young People Now*, 6 January. www.cypnow.co.uk

Mahadevan, J. (2011) 'Young people write to Cameron in defence of youth services', *Children and Young People Now*, 17 January. www.cypnow.co.uk

Moss Kanter, R. (1994) 'Collaborative advantage: the art of alliances', *Harvard Business Review*, vol. 72, part IV (July–August): 96–108.

Mulgan, G. (2005) 'Joined up government: past, present, future', in Bogdanor, V. (ed.) *Joined Up Government*, Oxford: Oxford University Press, pp. 175–87.

Smith, M. K. (2003) 'From youth work to youth development', *Youth and Policy*, 9, Spring, no. 79: 46–59.

Tyler, M., Hogarth, L. and Merton, B. (2009) *Managing Modern Youth Work*, Exeter: Learning Matters.

# 12  The management of faith based youth work

*Simon Davies*

This chapter focuses on the management of Christian youth work, within the context of local Christian faith communities. Historically speaking youth work in the UK has its pre-Albemarle roots in a religious and Christian motivated social concern (Davies, 1999). Despite this the Christian faith has certainly not been alone in influencing youth work. Most recently, the emergence of Muslim youth work, and an associated graduate level training programme,[1] reflects the growing awareness of what youth work, as a methodology, might have to offer the Muslim community in the UK. The Jewish faith also has a longstanding tradition of vibrant youth work, ranging from Jewish informal education and youth activities (Chazan, 2003), and youth movements (Rose, 2005).

This being the case, faith based youth workers, whether Jewish, Christian or Muslim, who have undergone professional training, would want to distinguish between activities that keep young people included in their respective faith communities, and those which work with young people engaging them in their respective ethical and social teaching, and exploring their own identity and wellbeing in contemporary society. This tension is connected to the way in which young people are thought about, and related to, by the faith community. Anxiety about 'losing young people' can lead to an atrophying of the educative character of youth work, and a very top-down, adult controlled curriculum. Youth workers in such contexts 'stand in the gap' – between generations, cultures and modes of education; to a certain extent they operate at the flux of the hopes of adults, and the aspirations of the young. This anxiety perhaps could be argued to be reflective of the broader attitudes of society towards the young; subject to the same moral panics (Davies, 1986; 2005).

Although an argument could be made for certain commonalities in the social and political experience of faith groups, it is simply not possible to generalize too much about the specific experience of 'management' across the whole sector. It is prudent therefore to limit the discussion of this chapter to the managing of youth work within the Christian sector, given that this both represents the majority of faith based youth work in the UK, and best represents the experience of the author. But it is hoped that those who are familiar with the management contexts of other faith communities may find some resonance with the following critique.

## Christian youth work

Youth work is one way in which the Christian church fulfils its purpose and exercises its moral and social responsibility within society. In doing so, it aims to be 'redemptive' of the people and structures it encounters. In this sense it shares its concern with the intentions of secular practice as it: *'represents an attempt to interfere in and, by some criteria, to "improve" or correct a given social order'* (Jones, 1985, in Levin, 1997: 25) and is also concerned *'in a broad sense [with] "wellbeing" but refers to some kind of collective provision which protects people's welfare'* (Spicker, 1995: 4–5). However, Christian youth work might at times make radically different statements about the *means* by which redemption in human societies occurs, and be divergent in its practice to include Christian spiritual disciplines and commitments (e.g. prayer, mediation, participation in acts of worship) as critical aspects of its work (Dean, 2004; Thompson 2007). It may also shift the *horizon of purpose* beyond the achievement of a particular material, physical or social state of affairs to a connectedness to ultimate purpose as understood by the Christian faith. Wellbeing then is understood to encompass the transcendent, as well as the temporal.

For the purposes of this chapter, the definition of Christian youth work that will be used will be that which is constructed through the convergence of:

- A concern with engaging with young people with respect to their holistic development – personal, social, and political – but also to their faith/spiritual development, where faith/spiritual development is understood to interpenetrate the former and relate (explicitly or implicitly) to the core Christian narrative (Butler and Butler, 1996; Moss, 2005; Nash and Pimlott, 2010).
- The core principles and purposes of youth work critically embedded in all that it does (Young, 1999; Jeffs and Smith, 2005; Roberts, 2009).
- The local church as the employment context of the worker, with youth and community work undertaken both within and outside of the faith community in the local geographical context.

## 'The community' and faith based youth work management

It is important to note that a significant proportion of funding for Christian youth work jobs derives from the charitable giving of members of the Christian community itself. These individuals are likely to live in the local geographical community, and possibly have children who attend local schools, clubs and associations. This means that the agenda and scope of the work tends to be set along the lines of particular 'local' concerns, based on these people's experience of living in a given area, and their commitment to their own children's, and their peers', circumstances.

In part this originates from what a Christian community is fundamentally aiming to be: *a community*. A community which brings together, by definition, a combination of *commonality* and *moral values* (Etzioni, 1995), as faith community members tend to not only be connected by geography and secular interests, but more importantly through their experience of faith, and their spiritual beliefs. The role of a Christian youth worker is therefore grounded in a potentially difficult but nonetheless intentional movement towards what Peck (1987) calls 'true community'. This process is one in which people move from 'being nice' through 'chaos' and 'brokenness' to a state of deep respect and true listening. This continually takes people more deeply into the everyday moral landscape of forgiveness, trust and moral responsibility outside of formal systems and controls. The community however, has a key role in shaping moral character and developing ethical literacy. This is simply because moral knowledge comes after choice and action in relation to *the other*, and it is 'community' which provides a repeated experience of these interactions and transactions (Byrne, 1999: 24).

Drawn from theological and historical sources, faith communities generally have an objective, rather than subjective view of moral values (e.g. the Ten Commandments), and this offers an ongoing framework within which 'the good' is debated, measured, pursued and realized. As a result, members of the faith community are engaged primarily in a moral project. Not that this approach to youth work is exclusive to faith based youth work, as there is some resonance with Young's (1999: 40–59) perspective that youth work is at least in part a moral, spiritual and philosophical project, of enabling young people to explore their own values in the context of living with others.

Habermas (1981, cited in Outhwaite, 2009) in his concern for the colonizing aspects of the state and the market, distinguishes between the two spheres of 'society' and 'community', describing them as the 'system' and the 'life-world'. He describes what amounts to the invasion of the latter by the former, an invasion that interrupts the communicative action that underpins the formation of the life-world (community). It is argued that the basis of healthy social life and human wellbeing is the life-world not the system. The 'system' replaces discourses centring on 'being' with discourses centring on 'function'. These functions are technical in aspect and ideologically oriented towards efficiency and productivity. As a result the organization which is constructed becomes a dehumanizing machine, as interaction, including language, takes on the character of the system.

Quinn (2003) reinforces this perspective, in identifying the socio-historical contexts that have contributed to the evolution of management. The culture of managerialism, with an emphasis on the technocratic qualities of managers, embodies this shift to the predictable fulfilment of predetermined outcomes. This is only really possible through a high level of control and the implementation of standardized processes. One needs a highly tuned and ordered system in order to achieve it. Therefore, as Western society increasingly becomes committed to rational, technocratic, mechanistic solutions – what Habermas (1963, cited in Outhwaite, 2009) identifies as an ideological commitment to 'scientism' – it is unsurprising that these values are evident in shaping thinking and practice in the management of social institutions.

However, with a genuine commitment to community, and an embracing of the 'life-world' as opposed to the 'system', there is a clear clash of cultures between the local Christian church and dominant managerial practices. Since the origins of such an ideological resistance are held by the faith community to have originated ultimately from a transcendent reality, and an historical tradition, they therefore carry more gravitas than that of the present social order. These commitments to 'becoming community' can therefore provide a point of resistance to the colonization of faith communities by the inherently ideological commitments of modern management, and consequently its practice.

## Leadership of Christian youth workers

It would certainly appear that the language of *leadership* is embraced more fully than that of management within the Christian community (Adair, 2001; Cocksworth and Brown, 2002; Croft, 2002; Pritchard, 2007; Walker, 2007). There is, by comparison, little literature that adopts 'manager' as a way of talking about particular roles in the church. Ways of leading within the Christian church have ancient historical roots of biblical origin. Croft (2002) identifies four modes of leadership that form the roots of these historical forms of leadership, namely: (a) one who champions justice, (b) one who is a wise teacher, (c) one who restores, and (d) one who rules and makes laws. Bringing the language up to date a little, immediately we can begin to identify these four dimensions in the leadership (and management) of faith based youth work, when re-described as 'centred on justice', 'committed to education', 'seeking to bring about a wholeness of being', and 'boundary setting'.

Croft continues to identify three principles which underpin Christian leadership, the first of which is that of servanthood, relating to the status, aims and exercise of leadership. In particular the concept of servanthood refers to the laying down of self for the sake of others, rather than seeking one's own advancement and recognition. Through the non-dominant exercise of power, the aim of leadership is to enable the community to excel by developing their own skills and fulfilling their own potential. Ultimately the desired transformation of those who are being led in this manner is that they in turn excel in their servanthood toward others; a kind of cascade of enabling.

Second, for Croft, the issue of *moral character* is uppermost in leadership. There is a desire for those who are exercising leadership to be recognizably trustworthy, honest, faithful, egalitarian and compassionate. This is simply the recognition that much, if not all, of human activity has a moral or ethical dimension, but it also reflects the primarily moral space of community. So being literate and attuned in this area is seen as a critical faculty for leadership in this context.

Third is the importance of *modelling the faith-life*. This essentially comes down to being an example of the 'good life' as defined by the Christian faith, in addition to being invested in spiritual disciplines such as prayer, reflection, solitude and meeting needs of the community. A parallel can be drawn here with secular notions of leaders as role models, as well as with Covey's (2003) concept of 'principle centred leadership' which places an emphasis on the moral character of the leader or manager as being the deciding factor in their success at the head of the organization. Although clearly Covey's is a secular notion based on fairness and justice and doesn't have any religious connotations.

Dantely concurs with this moral basis of leadership, arguing:

> Faith cause[s] a leader to actualize other human beings from a moral standpoint. Such an ethical actualization demands a moral way of interacting and engaging with those on whom leaders have impact and influence.
>
> (2005: 9)

Suggesting that this ethical orientation towards the other provides for a 'caring ethic', which he identifies as 'a spiritual activity that exudes faith in the continuous process of the humanization of men and women. [It is faith,] informed by a morality of care, that subsumes transformative leadership' (Dantely 2005: 10).

Cornel West (1988) in Dantely (2005), alluding to what he describes as the 'prophetic spirituality' which underpins the African American community, concludes that there is a deep need to 'ground the work of education in a context of *morality and meaning*, two concepts that seem foreign to this era' (2005: 15). As we have seen previously in this volume, whether looking at management theoretically in Chapters 3 and 4 or more practically in relation to issues of evaluation or supervision in Chapters 7 and 8, faith based youth work reminds us of the importance of 'value laden' rather than 'value neutral' leadership and management. Not of course that this has to be from a religious perspective; as McKenna et al. (2009) propose, the concept of wisdom, often seen as a 'spiritual quality', could be used as a meta-concept to evaluate management or leadership regardless of the context. They see 'wisdom' as a way to bring together (a) the logical/rational and the intuitive/subjective in the exercise of 'good judgement', (b) the integration of thought and action, and (c) knowing and seeking the inherent satisfaction of contributing to the 'good life'. They see an interesting congruence between the literature of spirituality and that of transformative leadership, both of which emphasize the ethical dimension, and manage with an emphasis on the organization's values and inspiring staff towards a vision. They lead 'through consent and commitment rather than through control and sanctions' (Ford et al. 2005: 84).

## Managing of Christian youth workers

As we have seen, Christian youth workers are being recruited to work in a particular community, and whilst having the remit of working with young people, they also are expected to fulfil a particular role in relation to that community. This role is characterized by a high degree of informality. However, being in a position of employment, on the contrary, implies considerable formality. As a result conflicts begin to emerge. How will the language and values of the profession cohere with notions of the Christian community? What kind of relationship does the rest of the faith community have towards the youth worker and how are the responsibilities of youth work to the wider community defined? It is not surprising that Richards (2005: 34) concluded that the reasons frequently cited for youth workers considering giving up were not the young people, but the organizational context of the work, and lack of understanding of their role as the main contributors. They also cited good supervision, supportive colleagues and a sense of personal fulfilment as those things that kept them motivated. It is to the supervision of youth workers that we will now turn our attention, before returning to some of these wider organizational issues.

### *Supervision of Christian youth work*

First it is important to recognize that a church leader (such as a pastor or vicar) is responsible for the oversight of more than simply the work with young people. They will have a responsibility to adults of all ages, perhaps especially the elderly, and be concerned with a variety of needs from the physically and mentally ill, to parenthood and bereavement. As a result this means that weighing up the needs of young people in the context of the needs of the wider Christian community is a difficult task. Second, it is quite possible they have little understanding of youth work (Richards, 2005) and are therefore unaware of the role of the youth worker in the personal and social development of young people. Third, they are unlikely to have had any experience or training in 'management' (unless they have moved from another professional field into church leadership) and will have little more than an intuitive grasp of management practices.

Given the previous emphasis on 'Christian leadership' and the wider development of the Christian community in the priorities of church leaders, it comes as no surprise that this profoundly affects the type of supervision afforded to Christian youth workers. Arguably the supervision of youth workers has a clear focus on, first, the personal or pastoral needs of those to be supervised, and second, it is likely to highlight the development of faith commitment and spiritual expression. Not that it is being argued that these are unimportant in the lives of Christian youth workers, or that support of these aspects is not required. But it is important to identify the bias in what is likely to transpire in the supervision process. As we saw in Chapter 8 on supervision, Kadushin's three essentials of supervision – of restorative, formative, and educative functions – provide an important check on the bias of the supervision; arguing that each of these must be present in effective supervision (Kadushin, 1992; Kadushin and Harkness, 2002).

Clearly, Christian youth work supervision focuses almost exclusively on the restorative element. Important implications arise out of this 'imbalance' in supervision, which ignores the educative and formative function. As a result there is a tendency to create 'lone rangers'. Youth workers who are supervised by people who have little or no understanding of the educative purposes, or processes, of youth work and are unable to offer direction to their work. For some, who have a specific need for feedback on the quality of their practice, perhaps those new to the role, or those who are recently qualified, it is likely there will be considerable frustration. But no doubt all youth workers would benefit from someone who holds a mirror up to their practice, and reflects back critical questions about 'what works' and how to improve it.

The increase of the training opportunities now available for youth workers who are Christians,[2] it could be argued, has had an impact on the experience of being supervised, and managed, and therefore exacerbated this issue. Professional training requires that youth workers demonstrate understanding and skills in 'managing others' (e.g. PNOS 5.2); the frame of reference is one primarily drawn from contemporary management literature, rather than the values and priorities emerging from the culture of 'church leadership'. A conflict is likely to be provoked by the different set of experiences in training and the frames of reference of church leaders in practice.

As a result of these a 'high-support/low directive' relationships, the supervisor may well believe that they are fulfilling their role of overseeing the youth worker (according to their values and priorities). They simply do not have the expertise to structure and to direct the youth worker's practice. This may be experienced by the youth worker as meeting with someone who appears to be uninterested in youth work, and unable to offer concrete direction. They also may not be able to offer any constructive or critical feedback on what the youth worker is actually doing. Do they even share the same 'success criteria'? This 'educational' aspect of managerial supervision is precisely what Kadushin identifies. It is also what may well be expected from professionally trained youth workers as being the central features of managerial supervision.

Interestingly, Kageler's (2009) research in both the United States and Europe clearly showed that Christian youth workers identified a poor relationship with supervisors (alongside isolation/loneliness, and an 'unnourished' soul), as one of the three main reasons for burnout. It is clearly problematic when supervision is cited as causing problems rather than alleviating them. Brown and Bourne (1996) argue that it is often more difficult to develop an effective supervisory relationship without any clear contract between participants at the outset. It would certainly seem to be the case that both church leaders and Christian youth workers must take some responsibility in renegotiating the content and function of those supervisory relationships, in order that effective 'managerial supervision' might develop both the youth worker, and the youth work.

The scope of supervision which emphasizes spiritual direction may begin to look much more like 'non-managerial supervision' or even nondirective counselling rather than supervision itself. For secular youth workers this personal dimension to supervision, free from any association to the work delivered, would be considered by some to be inappropriate territory; Adirondack (1998) might well refer to this approach as being symptomatic of the reluctant manager, one who avoids taking responsibility for the direction of the work and the need to address issues of practice directly. For others this may be an attractive prospect, particularly for youth workers who experience the current climate of managerialist supervision explored in Chapter 8. The creation of a safe space to explore and develop one's personal as well as professional self, without the demands of accountability, might come as a welcome relief.

## Organizational context of Christian youth work

In Christian communities there is often an almost self-conscious effort to understand what it is that those involved are trying to do, and be, together, both in the community context, and in relation to wider society. This kind of activity is the central purpose in Christian theology, as ultimately theology *'is the attempt by faith to understand itself, its object and its place in today's world'* (Hart 1995: 1). Christian theology therefore is an activity best described as: *'the disciplined and critical reflection of the community of faith upon the gospel entrusted to it'* (Hart 1995: 11). Christian communities therefore aim to live and to learn together, acting upon, or living out its core beliefs and values in ways that have integrity in the contemporary context. This rightly indicates that theology thus conceived is an active process, an embodied or *incarnated* business, including human agency and material, social and political realities, rather than being simply concerned with the metaphysical or the systematic organization of belief.

The youth work developed by a local Christian community, because of this free, voluntary invitation to intellectual, and practical, activity has the potential, in theory at least, to generate diverse and creative responses to young people's needs. This freedom of expression is contrasted markedly with the neoliberal managerial controls that have become so evident throughout secular youth work. This has led Smith to propose that:

> in the immediate future, youth work with its relational and convivial nature is more likely to flourish in non- or limited-state funded organizations. These include churches and religious bodies.
>
> (2003: 54)

But importantly it also demonstrates that the outcomes of youth work are not dependant upon the specific prescription and predetermination that the current managerial controls assume and demand.

At its worst, however, Christian youth work is a context where innovation, creativity and diversity is being crushed because of the weight of established tradition and culture. One of the reasons for this, and why Milson (1983) argues that churches fail to become seriously politically engaged, is that first and foremost churchgoers are primarily looking for the satisfaction of their own needs. Churches intend to be safe places to find healing, hope, meaning and purpose within the context of others who are seeking the same. Second, association with churches is often tinged with nostalgia, a security in the past, away from the troubles of the present (ibid.). This is perhaps the cost of having familiar sets of practices that individuals may have participated in, and that have remained largely unchanged, since their childhood. This consistent successful satisfaction of one's own needs, amongst others, is extremely important in terms of people feeling that they actually belong to a community, but it can produce an environment which can be highly resistant to change.

Christian youth workers stand in a unique position mediating the relationship between young people and adults in a variety of contexts; often 'standing in the gaps' between:

- The expectations and values of adults, and those of young people
- The expectations and values of parents, and their children[3]
- The practising faith of adults, and that developing in young people in the light of their own youth culture
- Those already belonging to the faith community, and those who do not
- The values, language and educational practices of professional youth work and those of the local church/Christian tradition.

The demands placed upon Christian youth workers by the requirements of such mediation, are pressurized and can produce stress, as well as lead to isolation and emotional exhaustion. The challenge for Christian youth workers within this context is whether they become facilitators of genuine interaction and integration, or merely become providers of specialist separate provision. Whilst the latter may satisfy the immediate need identified by adults to contain 'their' young people, and ensure they maintain a commitment to their faith community, it ultimately may not serve to enable the whole community to change, and enable young people to fully participate in the community according to their capacities as growing and developing human beings.

Ward (1996) shows that particularly within the evangelical tradition, Christian youth work has been hugely influential in the regeneration of the church. On reflection, the development of an active concern for another (at times culturally unfamiliar) group, which brings with it its own perspective, attitudes and priorities into the community, can serve to puncture nostalgia and awaken people to the needs of others in addition to their own. This may also bring about the questioning of the values and beliefs of adults, by the young, and leads to the re-examining, clarifying and reframing of commonly held beliefs. Whilst this questioning, in theory at least, accords with the fundamentals of any faith community, the more 'conservative' communities may not welcome such intrusions.

As we saw in Chapter 9 in the discussion of centre based management, youth policy has increasingly separated youth work provision from its community context, where the 'treatment' of young people is prescribed in an increasingly individualized manner through institutions and professionals. Christian faith communities potentially provide a context where intergenerational understanding can be fostered, and facilitate the genuine production of 'social capital' (Putnam, 2001).

### 'Calling' and the management of boundaries

Smith (1999) describes the notion of 'calling' or vocation as the dynamic congruence between an individual's identity, values and aspirations, and the occupation they choose. This has specific resonance and currency with Christian youth workers' self-definitions

(Richards, 2005). Whilst on one level this accordance between personal values and work life may bring a high degree of meaning and job satisfaction, a collapsing of the distinction between public and private life precipitates complexities and potential problems which require managing.

The following represent some of the important aspects of the context of delivering youth work, and are of particular relevance to managing personal and professional boundaries in Christian youth work

(a)  The geographic community that the work is *situated* within
(b)  The geographic community that the worker *lives* within
(c)  The field of the *personal* ('being' in relationship)
(d)  The field of the *professional* ('function' in the workplace)
(e)  The field of personally held *ultimate beliefs* (the 'faith' self)
(f)  The *faith community* (public expression of commonly held ultimate beliefs).

In secular youth and community work, whether statutory or voluntary, there may be complete separation of some, or all, of the above dimensions, and partial overlap of others. Indeed the professionalization of youth work, it could be argued, has encouraged the separation of personal life and professional work. However, as a youth worker within the context of a local church it is frequently the case that all of the above domains overlap to a considerable degree, and sometimes, in the case of particular elements, entirely so. For example, it is at least considered desirable, and at times a requirement, that a worker live within the geographic community they are working in. Sometimes it is the case that there is an expectation that the worker will make use of their own home as both an office, and a point of contact with young people. These realities can generate a situation where not only are boundaries blurred, but in some cases they cease to exist.

This principle finds resonance within Christian theology in the idea of *incarnation*; God becoming 'en-fleshed' and in so doing, associating completely with humanity in all its beauty and brokenness (Atkinson and Field, 1995). This has become a frequently cited principle for Christian youthwork: being there, associating as fully as possible with young people, entering their world so as to meet them where they are at (Ward, 1997; Passmore, 2003).

There is some similarity with the approaches taken by informal educators (Smith, 1994; Jeffs and Smith, 2005) who place an emphasis on 'being about': 'the aim, generally, is to be seen, to make and maintain contact with people' (Jeffs and Smith, 2005: 111). As well as 'being there [which] involves setting time aside for responding to situations ... being a shoulder to cry on in times of crisis involves taking steps to be contactable and in a position to respond' (ibid.). This approach helps to ensure that youth work practice is firmly located within the community and is responsive to their needs. There is also a real invitation here to cast off institutional priorities and step thoughtfully and intentionally into a positive place of practice that is well connected with young people and the communities they are a part of. However, as a result of the management practices adopted within Christian youth work this frequently generates lone rangers who head off into the sunset without a compass or a flask of water, with a shout of 'See you in 6 months for supervision!'

Richards (2005) comments on this intimate connection between personal motivation and identity on one hand, and professional practice on the other, suggesting that for

Christian youth workers faith, self and work become '*so interconnected that they cannot talk about them separately*' (2005: 47). This is clearly a 'double edged sword'; first it can lead to high levels of personal fulfilment and commitment that result from a real dynamic congruence between one's fundamental beliefs and one's working life. However, as one Christian youth worker clearly puts it:

> if our vocation is central to your sense of identity, then difficulties within your vocation are going to have an impact on your sense of self, and vice versa.
>
> (Richards, 2005: 141)

Booton has identified that: 'there are particular identifiable features of this work that positively encourage a complex of personal and professional problems which leads to distress and/or break down in some individuals' (1987: 99). He goes on to identify the stress that can lead to the youth worker becoming a 'casualty'. Not that this process is unique to faith based youth workers, but it would certainly appear that faith based youth workers are, if anything, more susceptible. Lake (1965) provides some very useful insights from the field of psychodynamics, and illustrates how the 'over-mixing' of the work self and 'personal self' can have serious implications for mental health and well-being. Where achievement, role and 'function' become the centre ground for status, purpose and nourishment in a person's life, rather than their 'being in relationship', then a cycle of seeking achievement in order to feel significant and valued can eventually result in mental health issues, and burnout. Walker (2007: 18) also identifies this cycle, but to a certain extent he sees it as being paradigmatic of being in a position of leadership and receiving affirmation from 'followers'. The crux of the matter here is that this potentially destructive cycle needs to be actively challenged in the self, which in turn necessitates the existence of safe and honest contexts for self-disclosure and self-discovery. Managing the personal/professional identity is an ongoing process, and quality line management is a necessary component in increasing youth workers' awareness of the boundaries of their responsibilities, and thereby attempting to maintain wellbeing. Although this might be taken for granted by those who work in other secular contexts, this issue is specifically highlighted because of the unusual level of personal/professional complexity due to the immersion in young people's lives and the community that is often expected of Christian youth workers.

Church leaders, however, are also caught in the same set of circumstances, and, given the emphasis on 'modelling' in the theoretical perspectives on church leadership indicated earlier, they can become part of the problem as much as they could be part of the solution. It is arguable that Christian youth workers would benefit from engaging in non-managerial supervision, spiritual direction, and pastoral care in order to thrive, rather than simply survive (Nash, 2006; Whitehead, 2010). In addition, many of the spiritual disciplines (e.g. De Mello, 1998; Foster, 2008) that have been developed within the Christian tradition are sets of practices and intentional relationships that can become a powerful personal resource for faith based workers, and help maintain wellbeing.

## Conclusions

It is quite evident that the management of Christian youth work is markedly different to that of secular youth work management and produces a different set of challenges.

It might even be the case that there is an ideological resistance to management within the employment context of much faith based youth work. More precisely, there is a resistance to some of the accepted forms, styles and values of management that might be encountered in the public or private sector, and have increasingly been incorporated into secular youth work. It is quite possible that Christian youth work could develop its management practices. Benefitting from clearer structures, and improving the management of its employment relationships, however, this resistance to management does aid the preservation of churches as communities of free participation, rather than organizations of controlled and directed action. It also helps preserve the 'goods' that religious communities have carried through the ages, and to maintain the belief that they have something significant and valuable to offer contemporary society.

For secular youth workers and managers the earlier discussions of faith based management provide a useful mirror in order for them to reflect upon their practice. The constraints of managerialism are clearly absent. Gone is the micromanagement and almost obsessive concern for accountability and control. Not of course that this lack of controls has necessarily led to poor youth work practice. Quite the contrary perhaps: youth workers freed from endless paperwork are enabled to fully immerse themselves in the life of the community and its young people.

However faith based youth work management does provide some challenges. The establishment of 'lone rangers' means the direction and focus of the work is almost entirely at the whim of the individual practitioner. The lack of a focus in supervision on the development of practice or issues of accountability, limits the potential of some Christian youth workers, and makes it difficult to identify and improve poor practice. Needless to say, as a result of the tendency to believe the grass is always greener, the Christian youth worker no doubt wishes they had a manager who paid much closer attention to their work, like those of their secular colleagues. Similarly the secular youth worker may well see the description of management in faith based youth work and wish they could experience such freedom. Indeed there is a degree of similarity between the original role of manager as 'advisor' identified by Davies in Chapter 1 and that of the 'church leader', in that both exercise little power over the priorities of the youth worker, although the original youth work advisors did have a specific interest in the development of practice, which it would appear the church leader does not always have.

There is also a tension within Christian youth work between progressive attempts to genuinely develop the community and embrace the lives of young people, who are not necessarily existing members of the church; and more regressive approaches which effectively deal with a closed community staid in tradition, resistant to change, and which merely ensure the adherence by young people to existing norms and values of the mainstream church. Another tension exists in the management of boundaries. On the one hand, youth workers are immersed in their community, experiencing the fulfilment of their calling with a congruence between their 'values and beliefs' and what they are able to achieve through their work. Paradoxically, through this absence of boundaries and lack of managerial support, problems can arise, and burnout result.

In short, Christian youth work management suffers from 'too little management' rather than its secular cousin which suffers from 'too much', although no doubt there is considerable debate as to which alternative individual youth workers would prefer. But there are many youth workers who have experienced the 'hand of managerialism' who would argue that their own managers could learn a lesson from the church leaders/ managers who have 'faith' in them and their practice.

## Questions for reflection and discussion

1   What lessons can secular managers learn from the approach taken by church leaders to the management of faith based youth workers?
2   Control or trust – should faith based youth work be made more accountable? If so how? If not why not?
3   Passionate and professional? – What are the advantages and disadvantages of vocational motivation?

## Notes

1  University of Chester.
2  E.g. the Centre for Youth Ministry launched an undergraduate programme, twinning professional training with theological education for Christian youth workers.
3  This is one of the unique features and difficult areas to negotiate in faith contexts, particularly because, as mentioned earlier, parents often are the primary funder.

## Further reading

Cosden, D. (2004) *A Theology of Work*, Milton Keynes: Paternoster Press.
Higginson, R. (1996) *Transforming Leadership: A Christian approach to Management*, London: SPCK.
Shirky, C. (2008) *Here Comes Everybody*, London: Penguin.
Walker, S. (2007) *Leading With Nothing to Lose: Training in the Exercise of Power*, Carlisle: Piquant Editions.

## References

Adair, J. (2001) *The Leadership of Jesus: And Its Legacy Today*, Norwich: Canterbury Press.
Adirondack, S. (1998) *Just About Managing: Effective Management for Voluntary Organisations and Community Groups* (3rd edn) London: LVSC.
Atkinson, D. and Field, D. (1995) *New Dictionary of Christian Ethics and Pastoral Theology*, Leicester/Westmont, IL: InterVarsity press.
Booton, F. (1987) 'Youth workers as casualties', in Jeffs, T. and Smith, M. (eds) *Youth Work*, Basingstoke: Macmillan, pp. 99–113.
Brown, A. G. and Bourne, I. (1996) *The Social Work Supervisor: Supervision in Community, Day Care, and Residential Settings*, Buckingham: Open University Press.
Butler, B. and Butler, T. (1996) *Just Spirituality in a World of Faiths*, London: Mowbray.
Byrne, P. (1999) *The Theological and Philosophical Foundations of Ethics*, London: Macmillan Education.
Chazan, B. (2003) 'The philosophy of informal Jewish education', in *The Encyclopedia of Informal Education*, available at www.infed.org/informaleducation/informal_jewish_education.htm (accessed 9 March 2011).
Cocksworth, C. and Brown, R. (2002) *Being a Priest Today*, Norwich: Canterbury Press.
Covey, S. R. (2003) *Principle Centred Leadership*, New York: Simon and Schuster.
Croft, S. (2002) *Ministry in Three Dimensions: Ordination and Leadership in the Local Church*, Darton: Longman and Todd.
Dantely, M. (2005) 'Faith-based leadership: ancient rhythms or new management', *International Journal of Qualitative Studies in Education*, 18(1): 3–19.
Davies, B. (1986) *Threatening Youth: Towards a National Youth Policy*, Buckingham: Open University Press.
——(1999) *From Voluntaryism to Welfare State: A History of the Youth Service in England, Volume 1, 1939–1979*, Leicester: NYA.

——(2005) *Threatening Youth Revisited*, available at www.infed.org/archives/bernard_davies/revisiting_threatening_youth.htm (accessed 9 February 2011).

Dean, K. (2004) *Practising Passion: Youth and the Quest for a Passionate Church*, Grand Rapids, MI: Eerdmans.

De Mello, A. (1998) *Sadhana: Christian Exercises in Eastern Form*, New York: Doubleday.

Etzioni, A. (ed.) (1995) *New Communitarian Thinking: Persons, Virtues, Institutions and Communities*, Charlottesville: University of Virginia Press.

Ford, K., Hunter, R., Merton, B. and Waller, D. (2005) *Leading and Managing Youth Work and Services for Young People*, Leicester NYA.

Forrester, D. (1997) *Christian Justice and Public Policy*, Cambridge: Cambridge University Press.

Foster, R. (2008) *Celebration of Discipline*, Sevenoaks: Hodder and Stoughton.

Hart, T. (1995) *Faith Thinking: The Dynamics of Christian Theology*, London: SPCK.

Jeffs, T. and Smith, M. K. (2005) *Informal Education: Conversation Democracy and Learning* (3rd edn) Nottingham: Educational Heretics Press. Kadushin, A. (1992) *Supervision in Social Work* (3rd edn) New York: Columbia University Press.

Kadushin, A. and Harkness, D. (2002) *Supervision in Social Work* (4th edn) New York and Chichester: Columbia University Press.

Kageler, L. (2009) 'Burnout among religious youth workers: a cross national analysis', Ph.D. dissertation, Nyack College, Nyack, New York (conference paper).

Lake, F. (1965) *Clinical Theology*, Darton: Longman and Todd.

Levin, P. (1997) *Making Social Policy: The Mechanisms of Government and Policies and How to Investigate Them*, Milton Keynes: Open University Press.

McKenna, B., Rooney, D. and Boal, K. (2009) 'Wisdom principles as a meta-theoretical basis for evaluating leadership', *The Leadership Quarterly*, 20: 177–90. Amsterdam: Elsevier.

Milson, F. (1983) *Political Education: A Practical Guide for Christian Youth Workers*, Exeter: Paternoster Press.

Moss, B. (2005) *Religion and Spirituality*, Lyme Regis: Russell House.

Nash, S. (2006) *Sustaining your Spirituality*, Y2, Grove Youth Series, Cambridge: Grove Publishing.

Nash, S. and Pimlott, N. (2010) *Wellbeing and Spirituality*, Y18, Grove Youth Series, Cambridge: Grove Publishing.

Outhwaite, W. (2009) *Habermas* (2nd edn) Cambridge: Polity Press.

Passmore, R. (2003) *Meet Them Where They're At: Helping Churches Engage Young People Through Detached Work*, Bletchley: Scripture Union.

Peck, M. S. (1987) *A Different Drum: Community Making and Peace*, New York: Simon and Schuster.

Putnam, R. (2001) *Bowling Alone: The Collapse and Revival of American Community*, New York: Touchstone.

Quinn, R. (2003) *Becoming a Master Manager*, Chichester: John Wiley.

Pritchard, J. (2007) *The Life and Work of a Priest*, London: SPCK.

Richards, S. (2005) 'The notion of vocation amongst Christian youth workers', Ph.D. dissertation, King's College, London.

Roberts, J. (2009) *Youth Work Ethics*, Exeter: Learning Matters.

Rose, D. (2005) 'The world of the Jewish youth movement', *The Encyclopedia of Informal Education*, available at www.infed.org/informaljewisheducation/jewish_youth_movements.htm (accessed 9 March 2011).

Smith, G. (1999) *Courage and Calling: Embracing Your God Given Potential*, Westmont, IL: Inter-Varsity Press.

Smith, M. K. (1994) *Local Education: Community Conversation Praxis*, Milton Keynes: Open University Press.

——(2003) *From Youth Work to Youth Development*. www.infed.org/archives/jeffs_and_smith/smith_youth_work_to_youth_development.htm (accessed 9 February 2011).

Spicker, P. (1995) *Social Policy: Themes and Approaches*, London: Prentice Hall/Harvester Wheatsheaf.

Thompson, J. (2007) *Telling the Difference: Developing Theologians for Youth Work and Youth Ministry*, Cambridge: YTC Press.

Walker, S. (2007) *Leading Out of Who You Are: Discovering the Secret of Undefended Leadership*, Carlisle: Piquant Editions.

Ward, P. (1996) *Growing Up Evangelical: Youth Work and the Making of a Subculture*, London: SPCK.

——(1997) *Youth Work and the Mission of God*, London: SPCK.

Whitehead, J. (2010) *An Introduction to Managing Yourself*, Cambridge: Grove Booklets.

Young, K. (1999) *The Art of Youth Work*, Lyme Regis: Russell House.

# 13 Managing in the voluntary sector
## The particular challenges of managerialism

*Ilona Buchroth*

Investigating the particular challenges in managing voluntary youth organizations, we need to first acknowledge the breadth and diversity of the third sector, which ranges from small neighbourhood projects to large, national and international bodies. These can be classified by their primary function, such as delivering services, mutual aid, or campaigning; or by their beneficiaries, their activity or even by the way they are resourced and controlled. However, one of the common features of voluntary, not for profit, bodies is how they are seen to contrast with public and private bodies on the basis of their governance, missions and values (Courtney 2002).

Appearances suggest that voluntary organizations often have a degree of freedom to be creative in the development of management structures and cultures. As such they have the potential to reflect the ethos and values of youth work, in being democratic, sharing decision-making and striving for a more equitable distribution of power. Their position as what became known under New Labour as the third sector, means they have a degree of independence and in theory at least can create ways of working that are separate and different from the dominant management paradigms. The voluntary youth sector, especially the smaller organizations, therefore, can find imaginative and egalitarian methods of working, both internally with staff and young people, as well as externally involving stakeholders.

However, voluntary sector management is becoming overlaid by concepts and approaches that have their roots in the public and increasingly the private sector; they are no longer immune from the dominant discourse of neoliberal managerialism. As a result, voluntary organizations need to negotiate their position in relation to the external context within which they operate. Most prominently, this context affects their accountability, governance, mission and independence. The resulting tensions pose a particular set of challenges to the sector.

### Managerialism and the new accountability

One of the main challenges to management within the voluntary sector arises out of the what Banks (2004) calls 'new accountability' and its resulting managerialism, with the increased requirement to work to predetermined outcomes and targets, as well as the need to adhere to extensive regulatory systems both internally and externally. Voluntary organizations increasingly find themselves in positions of having to work within frameworks, especially monitoring and evaluation processes, that mirror the requirements of the dominant funding bodies which '[were] applying lessons from the

"new managerialism" that had developed both in the private and public sector'
(Courtney, 2002: 30).

> Thus the growing external interest in the organization and management of VCOs
> [voluntary and community organizations] in the UK can be seen as closely linked
> with the policy trend over the last two or three decades to draw the VCO sector
> ever more closely into the mainstream of public services delivery. The more
> important the sector has become as an instrument of public policy implementation
> and the more governmental funding has been 'transferred' to the sector, the more
> the academic and policy spotlight has been thrown on the way individual VCOs
> and the sector as a whole are organized.
>
> (Cairns et al., 2005: 870)

## The impact of managerialism on the voluntary sector

This has caused a significant change in the dominant management paradigm within the
voluntary sector. From a position of a deep-rooted resistance to 'management' as a
concept primarily associated with the private sector (Handy, 1988; Drucker, 1992),
there now appears to be a well established culture of managerialism, as 'even small
community projects have begun to use the language of business plans, strategic choice,
quality outcomes, mission statements and competing stakeholders' (Batsleer, 1995, in
Courtney, 2002: 33).

However, the demands of new public management do not always rest easily with
some of the more informal methods of managing organizations and 'the growth in
managerialist culture can be seen as undermining voluntary organizations' distinctive
ethos and organizational features' (Osborne and McLaughlin, 2008: 76). Voluntary
projects, for example, attempting to adhere to internal democratic processes often
struggle with the lack of acknowledgement that these processes are time-consuming.
They are unlikely to respond adequately to tight deadlines without having to compro-
mise on their more collaborative and democratic approaches or, in some cases, their
non-hierarchical structures. Similarly 'task cultures', with their more egalitarian
approach of valuing skill rather than position, can turn into what Handy (1999) would
refer to as 'role cultures' with more clearly defined positions and lines of accountability.

As increased managerialism carries a significant administrative load (Cairns et al.,
2005) many organizations report that the resulting bureaucracy and focus on procedures and outputs with their corresponding reporting mechanisms can dominate the
work and divert time from direct work with young people (Banks, 2004; Davies and
Merton, 2009). Furthermore, dealing with these demands requires particular skills and
expertise that 'tend to value the manager more than the professional' (Tyler, 2009: 232).

Administrative demands therefore can take precedence over the needs of both users
and participants (Banks, 2004; Jeffs and Smith, 2008) as well as the values of agencies
(Carmel and Harlock, 2008; Diefenbach, 2009). These demands can then also pose a
threat to the professional autonomy of youth work practitioners as 'they control and
standardise activities previously within the sphere of professional judgement' (Banks,
2004: 40) whilst at the same time undermining the 'user-led' principle that is a fundamental aspect of many, especially local and grassroots, organizations.

Fulfilling the requirements of prescribed lines of accountability can cause the strategic management of the organization to become the domain of a select group of people

deemed to have the requisite skills and experience. These may even be specifically recruited, often increasingly from the private sector (Weinstein, 2003). Alternatively, especially in small organizations, there can be an over-reliance on paid staff, with the committee not fulfilling its function as a strategic and decision-making body. This can lead to a confusion of roles as paid staff can be managed by a committee that they have a professional responsibility to develop and support. Perhaps even more importantly, this 'professionalization' of management undermines the traditional governance of the voluntary sector, in particular in how organizations involve local stakeholders, beneficiaries and users.

> New Public Management ... sees accountability as upwards through contracts or outwards towards consumers. As such it stresses performance targets set by the centre and relies on consumerist forms of consultation.
>
> (Paxton and Pearce, 2005: 9)

The separation of management from the operation of the organization is reflected in the perception of youth work practitioner roles. As Banks (2004) observed, jobs that were previously designated practitioner roles had been redesignated into hybrid forms of 'practitioner/manager'. A further shift appears to have taken place in that it has become common that, especially large, youth organizations designate their most senior qualified practitioner as the 'manager' of the project, reflecting the increase in roles and responsibilities outside the traditional youth work domain. Consequently there seems to be a trend that managers of projects increasingly withdraw from youth work practice and concentrate largely on business and administrative functions and as a result can lose touch with face-to-face service delivery. This is a situation which, as we saw in Chapter 9, Bamber (2000) describes as the 'nightmare scenario' (see Figure 9.1 on page 116). This he argues is exacerbated in the voluntary sector where 'unlike middle managers in local authorities, they are often responsible for all the key functions of an organization ... which divert their key staff away from essential, front-line work' (Bamber, 2000: 8). This 'nightmare scenario' of youth work professionals increasingly subsumed under administrative and managerial tasks also has a direct impact on the professional development needs of the (often part-time, sessional) youth work staff.

### Funding patterns and effects of the contract culture

The effects of increased managerialism are amplified and further extended by the changes in the resourcing of the voluntary youth sector. Many voluntary organizations are now likely to have a portfolio of funding from a range of different sources, such as statutory grants, trust funding, contracts, service level agreements, etc. As Palmer and Randall (2002) point out, this broad funding base can give organizations a greater degree of flexibility and autonomy, whereas organizations such as independent charities, who do not receive government funding, are instead 'subject to the mood of the public' (2002: 27). 'Independence' is much more complex, however, than merely not being in receipt of government funding, as all funding sources pose a range of potential issues, demands and dilemmas that impact on the organization's operation, direction and future.

A significant impact on voluntary youth organizations derives from the altered funding regimes, often referred to as the 'contract culture', of commissioning or procurement. These funding streams are invariably associated with predetermined targets and outcomes and replaced grants that could support initiatives that were led by the needs and aspirations of their users. Instead 'services are now designed and initiated by governments and put out to tender on a payment for service basis' (Sercombe, 2010: 56).

It can be argued that these changes in funding regimes have substantially altered the position of voluntary organizations, undermining their independence and reshaping their operation in significant ways.

### Impact on governance

The professionalization of governance functions created by the New Public Management (NPM) paradigm is amplified by the complexities of the funding landscape that voluntary projects need to negotiate. Organizations managing a large portfolio of funding sources can find themselves in a position that they have to meet different sets of targets, work to different performance indicators and follow separate monitoring systems of a range of different funding bodies who could also be working to different time-scales. Meeting these demands can be labour intensive, both during the application process and in the subsequent monitoring and reporting. Moreover, the considerable expertise that is required to handle these demands may well put a strain on most voluntary committees. Perhaps not surprisingly therefore, a survey undertaken by the Joseph Rowntree Foundation revealed that three quarters of organizations reported that they were led by their paid staff rather than their management committees (Russell and Scott, 1997).

Alternatively, for the control to remain with the management board, the trustees or directors need to display a wide range of diverse skills and knowledge, such as business planning, knowledge of legal and regulatory issues, and quality assurance systems. Community and voluntary organizations are therefore 'under increasing pressure from governmental funders to improve their management and organizational systems – to build their capacity' (Cairns et al., 2005: 869). To ensure that these functions are fulfilled adequately some boards specifically recruit members with the required skills from other sectors. This is in keeping with the recommendation of a survey by the Institute for Philanthropy that boards should cast their net more widely and recruit from across a range of disciplines, skill sets and industries (Malone and Okwonga, 2011).

Although the professional boost to boards' capacity is likely to achieve the required compliance with externally defined standards (Kumar and Nunan, 2002) this approach is not without its problems. For example, external operational expertise can be separate from the understanding of an organization's missions and values. As one project worker explained:

> We had really competent people on our committee, who were very good 'bid writers', but you could tell they were not actually involved in doing the work, there wasn't the passion … so in the end I had to do the bid myself anyway.

On the other hand, as Weinstein (2003) observes, board members who are closely aligned to the organization's mission and values can become disillusioned and disenfranchised through the increased professional and 'business' orientation of the board, which increasingly focuses on functional management rather than on its raison d'être, feeling that their contribution is not valued (Jeffs and Smith, 2008).

A further layer of complexity and skewing of traditional methods of democratic control can arise out of the requirement to adopt new legal structures, as imposed by charitable trusts, government departments and other intermediaries providing funding to the voluntary and community sectors. Many, especially small, community based projects, have traditionally been legally defined as associations; that is, bodies which have no separate legal status to their constituent membership. This did not pose a particular problem for the majority of small organizations without paid staff and which did not own their own assets. However, as organizations acquire additional assets they may also need to consider incorporation.[1] Not only are incorporated charities more likely to receive public money (Clifford et al., 2010b), but some funders make incorporation an explicit condition (e.g. the government's Communitybuilders Fund).

The perceived or real additional responsibility arising out of incorporation appears to further skew the demographic of the board, where only those comfortable with taking on directorships and trustee status will put themselves forward. This, however, can become a difficulty; as a survey of key charities in Scotland confirmed, charities are facing an uphill struggle in retaining and recruiting trustees (SCVO, 2006). This is an issue that appears to be echoed by many smaller community based organizations who find it difficult to recruit the requisite number of trustees from their membership (Russell and Scott, 1997).

Some organizations appear to regard the growing 'professionalization' of their boards as an indication of the increased professional status and standing of the organization itself. Thus the involvement of other members can become tokenistic or marginalized, a trend that can become particularly pronounced with regard to the involvement of young people. A predominantly neoliberal perspective has shifted young people from being members with democratic rights (Jeffs and Smith, 2008) to clients and consumers of services whose rights and entitlements need to be safeguarded as a regulatory issue. If organizations 'see themselves as businesses then it is fairly easy and consistent to view young people as customers' (Jeffs and Smith, 2010: 68). Consequently young people are consulted as users and their satisfaction is recorded as are their needs and aspirations within the 'market'. Alternatively their participation is promoted under a 'citizens' agenda' and takes place primarily via formal and established structures, with a focus on predetermined agendas (Podd, 2010). Either way, this externalizes the involvement of young people as an operational aspect of management, rather than regarding young people's participation and involvement as the core business of a youth organization. In addition to the resulting democratic deficit, there are fewer opportunities for organizations to 'grow' their own workers and with that build on local knowledge and expertise – a valuable aspect of grassroots, developmental and sustainable youth work (Rogers and Smith, 2010).

### *'Locus of control' shifts to the state*

A significant amount, if not all, of an organization's work can become an extension of state services, which makes it difficult for users to distinguish between public and voluntary provision. Government funding sources are closely tied to government policy priorities, focusing for example on targeting hard-to-reach groups or responding to identified policy issues such as tackling teenage pregnancy rates, or antisocial behaviour. The expected targets and outcomes can seriously challenge the ethics, underlying values and principles of organizations. For example, organizations' practice is shaped 'by funding streams tied to policies concerned with the control and safeguarding of young people rather than their development' (Davies and Merton, 2010: 46) or they are expected to deliver centrally identified policy priorities which tend to focus on the perceived deficiencies of young people rather than their potentiality (Davies, 2005).

This challenges the professional autonomy of youth work organizations to respond to locally identified need (Banks, 2004) and it significantly shifts the locus of control from 'bottom-up' to 'top-down', potentially eroding one of the distinguishing features of the grassroots strand of the voluntary sector. As Sercombe notes: 'agencies are now effectively agents of government, still with some scope for autonomous action, but within increasingly prescribed limits' (2010: 56). As a result, the voluntary sector is unlikely to fulfil its wider remit of 'critic of the state' without risking withdrawal of funding (Osborne and McLaughlin, 2008: 76). Thus voluntary organizations 'that move into the public services provision role ... tend to lose their independence – their ability to decide for themselves their mission, goals, priorities, and operating methods' (Cairns et al., 2005: 877).

### Short termism and sustainability

The short-term nature of commissioned work and its dependency on meeting targets impedes long-term and strategic planning, compelling youth workers 'to work to short term deadlines when some more sustained results true to young people and their future development will only be achieved with a longer term framework' (Tyler, 2009: 240). Furthermore, many funding sources are offered on a 'pump-priming' basis, piloting innovative pieces of work without any clear strategy or support for their long-term sustainability, regardless of their success. Davies (2008) illustrates this with the example of the Neighbourhood Support Fund that was introduced in the late 1990s and generated an extremely wide range of highly successful projects, only a third of which, however, were funded into the second phase of the fund. This lack of continuity can pose some real challenges and be the source of much frustration, as one respondent in Davies and Merton's enquiry points out:

> [We do] high quality work only through external funding. We showcase it. The money ends, the work ends. There's no mainstream money. Only exceptionally do we get money for sustainable work, to support existing work. ... there's only continuity for young people by inter-weaving from one project to the next.
>
> (2010: 46)

Funding arrangements therefore highlight the paradox that the policy context is creating for youth work professionals: They have to be innovative whilst needing to adhere to previously set and planned activities (Tyler, 2009); they have to be entrepreneurial whilst being 'subject to centrally imposed initiatives, performance targets, close monitoring and audit which effectively constrain their opportunities for strategic choice' (Cornforth, 2004: 9). Although there is 'a mantra of joined up and "holistic" approaches to meeting individual needs there is an equal and sometimes conflicting imperative to fire specific bullets to hit and reach particular targets' (Williamson, 2007: 43).

Most funding streams favour time-limited, innovative pieces of work, and charitable trusts are generally unwilling to pick up time-expired projects, compensate for loss of state funding or indeed cover core costs. This can cause serious problems on an operational and structural level. Smaller organizations in particular, or those failing to address the implications of major growth and change (Scott and Russell, 2001; Cairns et al., 2005) can become disproportionately dependent on project funding, without sufficient core funding to provide a suitably stable infrastructure to manage or sustain those projects long term. Larger organizations, often benefitting from economies of scale, can be in a much better position to continue bidding for funds and increase their portfolio of funders (Jeffs and Smith, 2008). However, as Davies (2008) points out, there is therefore a possibility that charitable organizations, by providing the infrastructure for commissioned work, are in actual fact subsidizing state provision.

## Mission drift

A significant proportion of an organization's core time and resources can be spent chasing and managing contracts, thus reducing the time spent on carrying out the organization's original aims or mission. Thus 'a closer relationship with the state could bring discontinuity between "espoused" purpose and values and "operative" purposes and values' (Paxton and Pearce, 2005: 12).

Although pursuing funding opportunities for opportunistic reasons may not be entirely new, several studies (Scott and Russell, 2001; IVAR, 2006; Hutchison and Ockenden, 2008) suggest that the precarious financial situation organizations increasingly find themselves in leads to a shift in their remit, priorities and mission. For some organizations their original remit no longer fits current government priorities; others diversify their operations to become eligible for funding; and some find that funders' monitoring systems are ill-equipped to capture the outcomes – for example some of the 'softer' and longer-term or developmental outcomes – that they would consider to be closer to their overall mission (Hutchison and Ockenden, 2008). Decisions on whether to pursue new initiatives or to respond to new priorities often need to be made within tight deadlines that leave little time for reflection, let alone consultation or negotiation (Scott et al., 2000). There is growing evidence that some organizations diversify into activities and aspects of service provision for which they may not have the expertise (Davies and Merton, 2010), or the capacity and management structure to support (Hudson, 2010).

The dependence on the continuation of contracts for the survival of the organization, within a largely competitive environment and the resulting need to secure funding in ever increasing and overlapping cycles, can become an organization's main focus. Jeffs and Smith note that 'each bid presents a fork in the road', an ethical dilemma that asks: 'is it right for me to comply with the conditions that will be attached, or are they unacceptable?' (Jeffs and Smith, 2010: 57). They also warn of possible situations where: 'Ethical considerations become irrelevant and the business model provides the paradigm and profit the compass' (ibid.).

## Competition

The increasing need to compete for contracts can import values and requirements of the private 'for-profit-sector' into the voluntary sector (Courtney, 2002) where 'the language and realities of the market place (competition, tendering, cost centres), contracts and partnerships have become the norm' (Tyler, 2009: 237).

These competitive market mechanisms of funding bodies require voluntary organisations to demonstrate their effectiveness and efficiency using similar standards to the private sector, blurring the boundaries between private, public and voluntary sectors.

As voluntary organizations do not only compete with the private and public sectors but also with each other, the competitive environment can adversely affect the breadth of the voluntary sector. A mapping exercise of the voluntary and community sector confirmed that larger more professionalized organizations that can develop the infrastructure, and the expertise to meet these demands, are set to fare much better in this climate, and can 'squeeze out' smaller, community based organizations (NCVYS, 2008; Wylie, 2009). As a result some organizations grow in size and further increase their chances of attracting funding (Scott and Russell, 2001; Paxton and Pearce, 2005). A survey by the Third Sector Research Centre confirmed that the larger the organization, the greater the likelihood of drawing government funding. At least half of voluntary organizations with an income of £150,000 or more were in receipt of government funding, rising to two-thirds of voluntary organizations with incomes greater than £5 million (Clifford et al., 2010a). At the other end of the spectrum smaller organizations are shrinking and their likelihood of benefitting from government funding shrinks accordingly; for example only 0.4 per cent of all government funding was allocated to charities with annual incomes below £10,000 (NCVO, 2007).

## Negotiating the current climate

Research by Banks (2004) categorized practitioners' responses to the demands of the new management agenda under seven different points of a spectrum, ranging from an enthusiastic, uncritical embracing of the new demands to principled quitting, with various levels of partial compliance and resistance in between. A similar pattern of response can be observed in how voluntary organizations negotiate their external, predominantly neoliberal context. A recent enquiry revealed that 'many managers and some youth workers now regard targets and the head-counting which goes with them as normal and positive' (Davies and Merton, 2009: 14) as they provide workers with a focus that they felt they were lacking before. It appears that some organizations are therefore thriving, proud of their achievements in terms of meeting (often exceeding) targets and are adopting a proactive stance to new (funding) opportunities.

Others feel that 'targets were dominating their work and that only what could be measured was being valued' (Davies and Merton, 2009: 14), and that 'performance indicators and measurements ... [serve] to refocus practice on the indicators used, which may not actually represent valued, worthwhile or meaningful objects' (Smart, 2007: 77). Regarding these expectations as being incompatible with their mission and purpose, or indeed the principles of youth work, some organizations thus refuse to negotiate the tensions arising from the demands of the external environment. In one example from the northeast of England a project has decided not to accept or bid for any funding that requires them to target their work with young people.

Within the middle ground there are organizations which appear to be driven by what Tyler would call 'principled pragmatists' who 'will take care, in pursuing success, that their actions are not significantly compromising their values' (2009: 242). These are therefore attempting to find ways of strategically complementing their core business. As one project manager in Sunderland said: 'We always start with what we have got and see if we can find some funding to help with it; we don't go out looking for new things, turning ourselves into something we are not'. And there are others who develop strategies and methods to circumvent the restrictions placed upon them and who are seeking ways to interpret obligations liberally and creatively, attempting to meet the needs of young people within their prescribed frameworks.

As has been argued, the way organizations attempt to deal with these tensions, and the rationale they adopt for their position, can pose a wide range of ethical issues. For example, to accommodate outcome- and target-driven funding streams, the needs and aspirations of young people can be severely compromised, providing a challenge to the professional ethics of youth work professionals. It is also possible that the need of workers to maintain projects can supersede the social usefulness of an organization. Moreover, the heightened competition between voluntary sector organizations can serve to undermine a collective voice of youth work organizations and create a culture of distrust and secrecy (Jeffs and Smith, 2008). This is amplified on a micro level as successfully negotiating the funding landscape also often involves nurturing entrepreneurial skills and competitive values in young people, which can be seen as being at odds with the more egalitarian and co-operative values generally associated with youth work (Jeffs and Smith, 2008, 2010). Similarly, finding ways to 'creatively' interpret the conditions imposed by funders can be regarded as teaching young people the skills of 'playing the system', thus potentially further compromising the integrity of professionals. Thus 'engaging with ethical questions around funding and involving young people within that conversation is a central task for workers and agencies. Without it claims to moral authority wither away' (Jeffs and Smith, 2010: 69).

Resolving some of these ethical tensions therefore asks for a dialogical approach which might also require decentralizing the role of leadership (Senge, 1990). This is particularly relevant, as balancing the value base and ethical demands of an organization does not just rest with professional workers and their professional ethics. It is a matter for the organization as a whole; one that needs to go further than satisfying the most immediate and obvious need, such as the requirements of regulatory bodies. Cairns et al. therefore argue that capacity building needs to go 'beyond building "competencies" and skills in individuals' and allow 'space for [organizations] to identify and reflect on their own understanding of the organizational challenges they face and to develop responses which they themselves consider appropriate to their own circumstances' (2005: 881).

Fulfilling the democratic imperative implicit in grassroots organizations therefore requires organizations both to examine their success in more expansive ways and to involve their wider constituency. Strategic management does not then remain the prerogative of a small number of individuals, such as the board of trustees, management committee or management team, but needs to involve the organization at all levels.

Furthermore, as we saw in Chapter 7, the evaluation of an organization's success should be taken outside the paradigm prescribed by funding bodies and the external policy context. It should start from within, that is, from the organization's own values and mission, using these as a basis for developing a more participative and holistic approach to evaluation and ultimately influencing strategic planning. Rather than just maintaining organizations by evaluating their effectiveness and efficiency, a more comprehensive, developmental process would require organizations to ask more fundamental questions relating to why they engage in activities and whether they should continue to do so. The latter approach, sometimes referred to as 'double loop learning' (Argyris and Schön, 1978), can be regarded as an essential prerequisite for an organization to maintain its internal democratic structure as well as a dialogical relationship with its external context, which, it can be argued, is also a fundamental function of the voluntary sector.

## Volunteering, the voluntary sector and the 'Big Society'

Under the last New Labour government, volunteering, especially for young people, became the focus of a number of policy initiatives, initially through 'Millennium Volunteers' (WCVA, 2011), a national accreditation for young volunteers aged 16–25 launched in 1999. Volunteering featured prominently, as 'making a positive contribution' – one of the five key outcomes of the Every Child Matters (ECM) agenda (DfES, 2003) and volunteering also became one of the four challenges of Youth Matters (DfES, 2005). Despite some initial suggestions, volunteering was never made compulsory; however, 'the implicit assumption which continued to underpin policy initiatives … was that it was young people above all who had a duty to "do their bit" for society' (Davies, 2008: 124).

It was evident that politicians wanted to extend volunteering to a more diverse group of people, widening the volunteer base to make it an attractive activity for those people who were not traditionally involved. The Institute for Volunteering Research was commissioned to undertake a wide-ranging research programme drawing attention to the link between volunteering and a plethora of social issues, such as mental health and social exclusion (IVAR, 2004). The government-backed Russell Commission (2005) also presented 'a national framework for youth action and engagement … to deliver a step change in the diversity, quality, and quantity of young people's volunteering', for a society in which 'young people feel connected to their communities [and] seek to exercise influence over what is done and the way it is done' (Russell, 2005: 6). This was followed swiftly by the establishment of the youth charity 'V' which received considerable government funding to facilitate volunteering (CYPN, 2006).

As we shall see shortly, the concept of the Big Society has a distinctive emphasis on volunteering; however, this emphasis on volunteering continues to focus on its potential to promote a particular set of outcomes. That is, it frames volunteering as an investment in a social infrastructure that is designed to counteract the perceived fragmentation of local communities. Despite locating volunteering in the social capital domain, this conceptualization is, however, 'instrumental' and decidedly neoliberal, as these attempts to invigorate social capital are primarily concerned with an investment in social relations with 'expected returns' (Lin, 2002) as opposed to being seen as a 'social good' (Sandel, 2010). The coalition government's proposed National Citizen Service 'aiming to help 16-year-olds develop the skills and attitude to engage with their community and become active and responsible citizens' (Cabinet Office, 2011a) can be regarded as the most current example.

Voluntary involvement ceases to be embedded as a central element of an organization's structure which places the community centrally. It does not arise therefore out of the needs and concerns of volunteers, but becomes externalized as a targeted and quantifiable output in its own right. This, as Smart suggests, can lead to a situation 'where activities, advice and volunteering come to be widely understood as the objectives of youth work, to be consumed, easily evaluated, withheld, listed and controlled' (2007: 77). Especially in larger organizations these outputs, alongside harnessing voluntary input, are increasingly managed separately as a discrete section of an agency's work. However, separating the contribution of volunteers, coupled with the parallel separation of management and practitioner roles of professional staff, can become problematic. As explained earlier, it creates a democratic deficit, which becomes amplified by the lack of involvement in the identification of and responses to local issues. Harnessing volunteer effort primarily for the delivery of services constitutes essentially a one-dimensional involvement. It does not necessarily provide the basis for a sustainable commitment to local issues, which arguably can be regarded as the pre-requisite for realizing a 'Big Society' vision. Long-term engagement is often linked to a fundamental value base rather than based on instrumental reasons (Beierlein and Preiser, 2005).

Ensuring long-term engagement of volunteers therefore is not just dependent on maintaining or 'servicing' their contribution, by for example offering practical support, but greatly depends on an environment that allows them to reflect on their values and beliefs and actively engage with the issues that are the central concern of the organizations they work with (Buchroth, 2007). However, providing this kind of environment makes particular demands on the structure of organizations as well as the professionals involved. The central position of 'relationships' in this context is well documented, either as a prerequisite to 'grow local youth workers' with an investment in their locality (Jolly, 2010), or nurturing a sustainable culture of voluntary engagement (Buchroth, 2007). As Spence (2004) and Ord (2004) point out, meeting targets and outcomes cannot be separated from the relationships that need to be developed and maintained in order to achieve them.

## The 'Big Society'?

The 'Big Society' made its first appearance in the Conservative Party's manifesto for the 2010 general election. Although very loosely defined (a recent survey showing '63 per cent of people say they still don't know what it means' [Cartmell, 2011]), it has gained considerable prominence and appears to remain David Cameron's 'big idea' (Norman, 2010). What is clear however, is that the Big Society places a distinctive emphasis upon the voluntary sector, focusing on 'a society where people come together to solve problems and improve life for themselves and their communities ... [and] ... for every adult in the country to be a member of an active community group' (Conservative Party, 2010).

The 'Big Society' vision puts the voluntary sector into sharper focus with the expectation that 'social enterprises, charities and voluntary groups play a leading role in delivering public services and tackling deep-rooted social problems' (Conservative Party, 2010). A plethora of proposed new initiatives is being developed to assist with implementing the 'Big Society' vision whilst also attempting to remove some of the perceived barriers that might hamper the voluntary sector generally. For example in December 2010 a new 'Barrier Busting Service' was announced by the decentralization minister, Greg Clark, allowing councils, community groups, local institutions and individuals to overcome bureaucracy and 'get things done in their neighbourhood' (Cabinet Office, 2010). A new Big Society De-regulation Taskforce aims to make it easier to run charities, voluntary groups and social enterprises by reducing bureaucratic burdens, and a 'Community Organizers' programme is being introduced to identify, train and support 5,000 people who want to make a difference to their community (www.cabinetoffice.gov.uk/content/big-society-overview).

However, these new and potentially supportive developments need to be viewed in the context of the comprehensive spending review of the coalition government, whose 'top priority is reducing the budget deficit, which was £156 billion in 09/10' (Webb and Allen, 2010). Although some additional financial support is being made available through, for example, the one-year transition funding that third sector organizations can bid for to assist with preparing for a tighter funding regime, or the announcement of the 'Big Society Bank', it is highly unlikely that these measures can balance out the effects of the comprehensive spending review cuts on the sector overall (NCVYS, 2010). Concerns about the impact of cuts on the realization of the 'Big Society' vision are gaining momentum from a wide range of perspectives, especially from infrastructure organizations supporting the third sector: Dame Elizabeth Hoodless, the retiring executive director of the Council for Voluntary Services, criticized the lack of strategy behind the 'Big Society' vision and pointed out that cuts were 'destroying volunteering' and were 'making it harder for people to do more in their communities' (BBC, 2011). These sentiments were echoed by Justin Davis Smith, chief executive of the charity Volunteering England, who, although supporting the 'Big Society' in principle, observed a 'disconnect between [the 'Big Society'] and the reality, where numerous organizations were having their capacity to deliver, to recruit more, to train, to support their volunteers, taken away from them' (ibid.).

As a result it may be argued that rather than strengthening the third sector, spending cuts could increase the burden on voluntary organizations to deliver the services that are being lost in the public sector. Moreover, job losses can adversely affect local infrastructures that are needed to harness and support the kind and size of voluntary effort that the 'Big Society' seems to suggest. Furthermore, however loosely defined, the 'Big Society' vision seems to suggest a more localized approach to decision-making and the delivery of services, and indeed, as Faiza Choudary, policy director for the National Council for Voluntary Youth Services, points out, 'small voluntary organizations are already delivering the big society vision' (quoted in Watson, 2010). Despite small organizations' arguably central position within 'Big Society' developments, they are the most dependent on public funds, are least likely to have reserves and are thus even more vulnerable in the current economic climate.

It could be argued that the lack of a clear definition of the 'Big Society' potentially offers opportunities for the voluntary sector to negotiate new meanings and positions. However, whether the most vulnerable, small, local organizations will survive in the short term to contribute to the debate is questionable. As core funding sources dry up, larger third sector players, those best placed to weather the storm, could increasingly displace those smaller organizations in the scramble to secure contracts aimed at meeting statutory sector agendas. If the current government allows this to happen, it will arguably preside over the demise of the organizations which are best placed to deliver on the 'Big Society' agenda. An effective campaign to highlight the need for an independent, vibrant, diverse, devolved, as well as well funded, third sector may be the only way that the imbalances set out above can be rectified. Such an effort, led by the larger national and regional third sector infrastructure and intermediary bodies, could begin to turn around a civil society policy environment which may otherwise destroy the very foundations that the 'Big Society' vision aims to develop. Without sufficient backing, the accusation that Cameron, in his construction of the 'Big Society', is putting 'words to work' (Garrett 2009: 3), appears correct and his 'vision' is merely a smokescreen for an ideological assault on 'welfarism'.

## Conclusion

As has been demonstrated, the breadth, scope and impact of voluntary sector youth organizations is shaped significantly by the external context which they need to negotiate. The complex demands imposed by managerial norms and funding patterns affect voluntary youth organizations' ability to respond to local issues as they increasingly need to meet targets and outcomes that are determined by external funding regimes. Furthermore, organizations have become more professionalized, which works to the detriment of smaller organizations and can weaken their grassroots involvement and affect the breadth and depth of the sector itself. A government emphasis on volunteering, conceptualized 'instrumentally' is at least 'once removed' from the community within which it is located. Furthermore, despite appearances that the 'Big Society' could provide a reinvigoration of the voluntary sector, there is little substantive evidence within its formulation to provide any hope that it is anything other than a neoliberal smokescreen for an ideological assault on a wide range of public sector provision, including youth work.

## Questions for reflection and discussion

1   Are small volunteer-led organizations the best way of meeting local needs? In what other ways can those needs be met, whilst retaining local involvement and accountability to both the local community and to funders?
2   How can local mutual support be mobilized in the current climate of community organizers – how will they operate and to whose ultimate agenda?
3   Are social enterprises a new way forward or a betrayal of bottom-up community activism?
4   How can central public funding be detached from quantitative output measures whilst still ensuring public accountability?
5   What are the prospects for the 'Big Society'? Is a vibrant voluntary sector plausible?

## Note

1   I.e. to create a legal entity that is separate from its members.

## Further reading

Barnard, H. (2010) *Big Society Cuts and Consequences: A Thinkpiece*, available at: www.cass.city. ac.uk/research-and-faculty/centres/cass-centre-for-charity-effectiveness/resources/thought-pieces
Davies, B. (2008) *The New Labour Years: A History of the Youth Service in England, Volume 3, 1997–2007*, Leicester: The National Youth Agency, chapters 7–9.
Jeffs, T. and Smith, M. K. (2010) 'Resourcing youth work: dirty hands and tainted money', in Banks, S. (ed.) *Ethical Issues in Youth Work*, Abingdon: Routledge, pp. 53–73.
Tyler, M. (2009) 'Managing the tensions', in Wood, J. and Hine, J. (eds) *Work with Young People: Theory and Policy for Practice*, London: Sage, pp. 233–46.
Wylie, T. (2009) 'Youth work and the voluntary sector', in Wood, J. and Hine, J. (eds) *Work with Young People: Theory and Policy for Practice*, London: Sage, pp. 202–12.

## References

Argyris, C. and Schön, D. (1978) *Organizational Learning: A Theory of Action Perspective*, Reading, MA: Addison-Wesley.

Bamber, J. (2000) 'Managing youth work in Scotland: a diversionary tale', *Youth and Policy*, Summer, no. 68: 5–18.

Banks, S. (2004) *Ethics, Accountability and the Social Professions*, Basingstoke: Palgrave Macmillan.

Banks, S. (ed.) (2010) *Ethical Issues in Youth Work*, Abingdon: Routledge.

BBC (2011) 'Cuts "destroying big society" concept, says CSV head', www.bbc.co.uk/news/uk-politics-12378974 (accessed 7 February 2011).

Beierlein, C. and Preiser, S. (2005) 'Gesellschäftliches Engagement', *Report Psychologie*, 30(5): 210–17.

Buchroth, I. (2007) 'Motivational and Situational Discourses in Collective Community Action', unpublished Ed.D. thesis, Durham University.

Cabinet Office (2010) *Tackling Bureaucracy in Local Communities*, www.cabinetoffice.gov.uk/news/tackling-bureaucracy-local-communities (accessed 7 March 2011).

——(2011a) *Government Puts Big Society at Heart of Public Sector Reform*, www.cabinetoffice.gov.uk/news/big-society-heart-public-sector-reform (accessed 3 March 2011).

——(2011b) *Big Society Overview*, www.cabinetoffice.gov.uk/content/big-society-overview (accessed 7 March 2011).

Cairns, B., Harris, M. and Young, P. (2005) 'Building the capacity of the voluntary nonprofit sector: challenges of theory and practice', *International Journal of Public Administration*, 28: 869–85.

Carmel, E. and Harlock, J. (2008) 'Instituting the third sector as a governable terrain: partnerships, procurement and performance in the UK', *Policy and Politics*, 36(2): 155–171.

Cartmell, M. (2011) 'Almost two-thirds of public baffled by David Cameron's "Big Society"', www.prweek.com/news/bulletin/UKDaily/article/1051960/?DCMP=EMC-CONUKDaily (accessed 28 January 2011).

Clifford, D, and Backus, P. (2010a) 'Are big charities becoming increasingly dominant? Tracking charitable income growth 1997–2008 by initial size', Third Sector Research Centre (TSRC) Working Paper 38. Birmingham: TSRC.

Clifford, D., Geyne Rajme, F. and Mohan, J. (2010b) 'How dependent is the third sector on public funding? Evidence from the National Survey of Third Sector Organizations', Third Sector Research Centre (TSRC) Working Paper 45. Birmingham: TSRC.

Communitybuilders Fund (2011) available at www.communitybuildersfund.org.uk/index.php?id=396 (accessed 8 March 2011).

Conservative Party (2010) *Conservative Party Manifesto* www.conservatives.com/Policy/Manifesto.aspx (accessed 3 March 2011).

Cornforth, C. (2004) 'The governance of co-operatives and mutual associations: a paradox perspective', *Annals of Public and Co-operative Economics*, 75(1): 11–32.

Courtney, R. (2002) *Strategic Management for Voluntary Nonprofit Organizations*, London: Routledge.

CYPN (2006) 'Analysis: Practice – Russell Commission – Charity strives to bring in a million volunteers', www.cypnow.co.uk/news/757533/Analysis-Practice-Russell-Commission-Charity-strives-bringing-million-volunteers/ (accessed 4 March 2011).

Davies, B. (2005) 'Youth work: a manifesto for our times', *Youth and Policy*, Summer, no. 88: 5–27.

——(2008) *The New Labour Years: A History of the Youth Service in England, Volume 3, 1997–2007*, Leicester: National Youth Agency.

Davies, B. and Merton, B. (2009) 'Squaring the circle? The state of youth work in some children and young people's services', *Youth and Policy*, Summer, no. 103: 5–24.

——(2010) *Straws in the Wind: The State of Youth Work Practice in a Changing Policy Environment (Phase 2)*, Leicester: DeMontfort University.

DfES (2003) *Every Child Matters*, London: HMSO.

——(2005) *Youth Matters*, London: HMSO.

Diefenbach, T. (2009) 'New public management in public sector organizations: the dark sides of managerialistic enlightenment', *Public Administration*, 87(4): 892–909.

Drucker, P. F. (1992) *Managing the Nonprofit Organization: Principles and Practices*, Oxford: Butterworth-Heinemann.

Garrett, P. M. (2009) *'Transforming' Children's Services? Social Work, Neoliberalism and the 'Modern' World*, Maidenhead: McGraw-Hill Education/Open University Press.

Handy, C. (1988) *Understanding Voluntary Organizations*, London: Penguin.

——(1999) *Understanding Organisations*, London: Penguin.

Hudson, S. (2010) 'Mission drift on the rise as charities go where the money is', *Third Sector Online*, 20 December, www.thirdsector.co.uk/news/Article/1047274/Mission-drift-rise-charities-go-money-is/ (accessed 8 March 2011).

——(2011) 'Almost half of trustees "appointed through personal recommendation"', *Third Sector Online*, 23 February, www.thirdsector.co.uk/channels/Management/Article/1056500/Almost-half-trustees-appointed-personal-recommendation/ (accessed 9 March 2011).

Hutchison, R. and Ockenden, N. (2008) 'The impact of public policy on volunteering in community-based organizations', in *Institute for Volunteering Research/Institute for Voluntary Action Research*. Available at www.ivr.org.uk/NR/rdonlyres/B796F0A0-632F-4D0E-B2C9-24AA3E6F7859/0/Impact_report_final.pdf

Institute for Volunteering Research (2004) *Volunteering for All? Exploring the Link Between Social Exclusion and Volunteering*, London: Volunteering England.

IVAR (2006) *Servants of the Community or Agents of Government? The Role of Community-Based Organizations and Their Contribution to Public Services Delivery and Civil Renewal*, Final report for bassac, London: IVAR.

Jeffs, T. and Smith, M. K. (2008) 'Valuing youth work', *Youth and Policy*, Summer/Autumn, no. 100: 277–203.

——(2010) 'Resourcing youth work: dirty hands and tainted money', in Banks, S. (ed.) *Ethical Issues in Youth Work*, Abingdon: Routledge, pp. 53–73.

Jolly, J. (2010) 'Local youth work', in Rogers, A. and Smith M. K. (eds) *Journeying Together: Growing Youth Work and Youth Workers in Local Communities*, Lyme Regis: Russell House Publishing, pp. 1–12.

Kumar, S. and Nunan, K. (2002) *Strengthening the Governance of Small Community and Voluntary Organizations*, York: Joseph Rowntree Foundation.

Lin, N. (2002) *Social Capital: A Theory of Social Structure and Action*, Cambridge: Cambridge University Press.

Malone, D. and Okwonga, M. (2011) *The State of UK Charity Boards: A Quantitative Analysis*, London: Institute for Philanthropy.

NCVO (2007) *The UK Voluntary Sector Almanac 2007*, London: NCVO.

NCVYS (National Council for Voluntary Youth Services) (2008) *Every Organisation Matters: Mapping the Children and Young People's Voluntary and Community Sector*, London NCVYS.

——(2010) *Comprehensive Cuts: Report on Funding Changes in the Voluntary and Community Youth Sector*, London NCVYS.

Norman, J. (2010) *The Big Society: The Anatomy of the New Politics*, Buckingham: University of Buckingham Press.

Office for Civil Society, Cabinet Office (2010) 'Building a stronger civil society: a strategy for voluntary and community groups, charities and social enterprises', www.cpa.org.uk/cpa_documents/building_stronger_civil_society.pdf (accessed 3 March 2011).

Ord, J. (2004) 'Curriculum debate: the Youth Work Curriculum as process, not as outcome or output to aid accountability', *Youth and Policy*, Autumn, no. 85: 53–69.

Osborne, S. P. and McLaughlin, K. (2008) 'The study of public management in Britain: public service delivery and its management', in Kickert, W. (ed.) *The Study of Public Management in Europe and the US: A Comparative Analysis of National Distinctiveness*, London: Routledge, pp. 70–98.

Palmer, P. and Randall, A. (2002) *Financial Management in the Voluntary Sector*, London: Routledge.

Paxton, W. and Pearce, N. (2005) 'The voluntary sector and the state', in Paxton, W. Pearce, N. P., Unwin, J. and Molyneux, P. (eds) *The Voluntary Sector Delivering Public Services: Transfer or Transformation?* York: Joseph Rowntree Foundation, pp. 3–27.

Podd, W. (2010) 'Participation', in Batsleer, J. and Davies, B. (eds) *What Is Youth Work?* Exeter: Learning Matters, pp. 20–32.

Rogers, A. and Smith, M. K. (eds) (2010) *Journeying Together: Growing Youth Work and Youth Workers in Local Communities*, Lyme Regis: Russell House Publishing

Russell, I. M. (2005) *A National Framework for Youth Action and Engagement* (Report of the Russell Commission) London: HMSO.

Russell, L. and Scott, D. (1997) *The Impact of the Contract Culture on Volunteers*, York: Joseph Rowntree Foundation.

Sandel, M. (2010) *The 2009 Reith Lectures*, available at downloads.bbc.co.uk/.../20090609_there-ithlectures_marketsandmorals.rtf (accessed 4 April 2011).

Scott, D. and Russell, L. (2001) 'Contracting: the experience of service delivery agencies', in Harris, H. and Rochester, C. (eds) *Voluntary Organisations and Social Policy in Britain: Perspective on Change and Choice*, Basingstoke: Palgrave, pp. 49–63.

Scott, D., Alcock, P., Russell, L. and Macmillan, R. (2000) *Moving Pictures: Critical Issues for Voluntary Action*, York: Joseph Rowntree Foundation.

SCVO (2006) 'Red-tape and fear of role creating charity board member crisis', www.scvo.org.uk/tfn/news/red-tape-and-fear-of-role-creating-charity-board-member-crisis/ (accessed 10 March 2011).

Senge, P. (1990) *The Fifth Discipline: The Art and Practice of the Learning Organization*, London: Random House.

Sercombe, H. (2010) *Youth Work Ethics*, London: Sage.

Smart, S. (2007) 'Informal education, informal control? What is voluntary youth work to make of self-assessment?' *Youth and Policy*, Spring, no. 95: 73–82.

Spence, J. (2004) 'Targeting, accountability and youth work practice', *Practice: A Journal of the British Association of Social Workers*, 16(4): 261–72.

Tyler, M. (2009) 'Managing the tensions', in Wood, J. and Hine, J. (eds) *Work with Young People: Theory and Policy for Practice*, London: Sage, pp. 233–46.

Watson, R. (2010) 'Small charities bear the brunt of cuts despite big society pledge', in *Children and Young People Now*, 10 August. www.cypnow.co.uk

WCVA (2011) www.wcva.org.uk/volunteering/index.cfm?sub=8anddisplay_sitetextid=106 (accessed 4 March 2011).

Webb, D. and Allen, G. (2010) 'Background to 2010 spending review', House of Commons library. www.parliament.uk/briefingpapers/commons/lib/research/briefings/snep-05674.pdf (accessed 4 March 2011).

Weinstein, J. (2003) 'Master and servant: the myth of equal partnership between the voluntary and statutory sectors', in Leathard, A. (ed.) *Interprofessional Collaboration: From Policy to Practice in Health and Social Care*, Hove: Brunner-Routledge, pp. 249–61.

Williamson, H. (2007) 'Youth work and the changing policy environment for young people', in Harrison, R., Benjamin, C., Curran, S. and Hunter, R. (eds) *Leading Work with Young People*, London: Sage/Open University Press, pp. 34–49.

Wylie, T. (2009) 'Youth work and the voluntary sector', in Wood, J. and Hine, J. (eds) *Work with Young People: Theory and Policy for Practice*, London: Sage, pp. 202–12.

# Index